Effect Of Integrated Yoga Among Police Men

D1731259

By:
Ramesh P.

TABLE OF CONTENTS

TITLE	Page. No

Table of Contents	i
List of Tables	iv
List of Figures	v
List of Symbols and Abbreviation	vii

CHAPTER

1	**INTRODUCTION**	**1-15**
	1.1 Introduction	1
	1.2 Yoga	2
	1.3 Yoga for Policeman	3
	1.4 Integrated Yoga Module	3
	1.4.1 Asana	3
	1.4.2 Kriyas	4
	1.5 Benefits of Yoga	5
	1.6 Reason of the selection of topic	5
	1.7 Statement of the Problem	6
	1.8 Research Questions	6
	1.9 Assumptions	7
	1.10 Delimitations	7
	1.11 Limitations	9
	1.12 Hypotheses	10
	1.13 Significance of the Study	12

TABLE OF CONTENTS (Contd.,)

	1.14 Definition of the Operational Terms	12
	1.15 Organization of the Dissertation	14
II	**REVIEW OF RELATED LITERATURE**	16-55
	2.1 Introduction	16
	2.2 Studies on integrated Yoga Module	17
	2.3 Summary of the Literature	54
III	**METHODOLOGY**	56-68
	3.1 Introduction	56
	3.2 Selection of Subjects	56
	3.3 Selection of Variables	57
	3.4 Selection of Tests	58
	3.5 Orientation to the Subjects	58
	3.6 Competency of the Tester	59
	3.7 Reliability of the Instruments	59
	3.8 Reliability of the data	59
	3.9 Pilot study	60
	3.10 Training programme	61
	3.11 Collection of Data	62
	3.12 Administration of Tests	62
	3.13 Experimental Design	67
	3.14 Statistical Technique	68
	3.15 Summary	68

TABLE OF CONTENTS (Contd.,)

IV	ANALYSIS AND INTERPRETATIONS OF THE DATA	69-104
	4.1 Introduction	69
	4.2 Analysis of Data –Part I	70
	4.3 Analysis of Data – Part II	81
	4.3.1 Assumptions Tests	81
	4.3.2 Results of Analysis of Covariance (ANCOVA)	84
	4.4 Discussion on Findings	102
V	SUMMARY, CONCLUSION AND RECOMMENDATIONS	105-108
	5.1 Summary	105
	52 Conclusions	106
	5.3 Recommendations for Future Researcher	108
	REFERENCES	109-120

LIST OF TABLES

TABLE	TITLE	PAGE
3.1	Selection of tests	58
3.2	Intra class co-efficient on selected variables	60
4.1	Paired sample 't' test of experimental group on selected dependent variables	70
4.2	Paired sample 't' test of control group on selected dependent variables	73
4.3	Levene's test of equality of error variances on selected variables among experimental and control groups	82
4.4	Testing the significance of the regression of post test on pre test of selected variables	83
4.5	Analysis of covariance computed for experimental and control group for cardio vascular endurance	84
4.6	Analysis of covariance computed for experimental and control group for muscular endurance	87
4.7	Analysis of covariance computed for experimental and control group for resting pulse rate	90
4.8	Analysis of covariance computed for experimental and control group for breath holding time	93
4.9	Analysis of covariance computed for experimental and control group for stress	96
4.10	Analysis of covariance computed for experimental and control group for self confidence	99

LIST OF FIGURES

FIGURE	TITLE	PAGE
4.1	Mean values of Pre-test and post-test of cardiovascular endurance on experimental and control groups	75
4.2	Mean values of Pre-test and post-test of Muscular endurance on experimental and control groups.	76
4.3	Mean values of Pre-test and post-test of resting heart rate on experimental and control groups.	77
4.4	Mean values of Pre-test and post-test of breath holding time on experimental and control groups.	78
4.5	Mean values of Pre-test and post-test of Stress on experimental and control groups.	79
4.6	Mean values of Pre-test and post-test of Self-confidence on experimental and control groups.	80
4.7	Adjusted post test mean values of Experimental group and control group on cardio vascular endurance.	86
4.8	Adjusted post test mean values of Experimental group and control group on muscular endurance.	88
4.9	Analysis of covariance computed for experimental and control group for resting pulse rate	91

4.10   Adjusted post test mean values of Experimental group and control group on breath holding time.   94

4.11   Adjusted post test mean values of Experimental group and control group on Stress.   97

4.12   Adjusted post test mean values of Experimental group and control group on Self-confidence.   100

LIST OF SYMBOLS AND
ABBREVIATION USED

IYM   -   INTEGRATED YOGA MODULE

ASCI   -   AGNIHOTHRIS SELF CONFIDENCE INVENTORY

ANCOVA   –   ANALYSIS OF CO-VARIANCE

SPSS   -   STATISTICAL PACKAGE FOR SOCIAL SCIENCE

Ho   -   NULL HYPOTHESIS

H1   -   RESEARCHER'S HYPOTHESIS

DF   –   DEGREES OF FREEDOM

CVE   –   CARDIO VASCULAR ENDURANCE

F   -   F RATIO

Chapter I

INTRODUCTION

1.1 Introduction

The Police Force of Tamil Nadu is recognized among the most efficient and best in the country. It has a commendable track record, not only in the maintenance of law and order, but also in assisting the community whenever the need has arisen. While remaining people-friendly, the Police Force has also been effective in countering anti-social activities. Policing has become more people-centered societal effort. Regular activity, fitness and exercise, are critical for health and well-being of people of all ages. Research shows that everyone, young or old can benefit from regular exercise, either vigorous or moderate (Tamil Nadu Police Archives, 2007). Tamil Nadu Police Department is the primary law enforcement agency of the entire state of Tamil Nadu, India. It is over 150 years old and is the fifth largest state police force in India. Tamil Nadu have a police-population ratio of 1:632. For administrative purposes, the state has been divided into four police zones – North, South, West and Central, each headed by an Inspector General of Police (Tamil Nadu Police Archives, 2007)

Police work can vary from routine office procedures to highly demanding situations, e.g arrest tasks, in which the circumstances are often unpredictable Policemen frequently have to deal with violent people Therefore police work places special demands on the quality and quantity of a policeman's psychological and physiological work capacity The need for policemen to be physically fit is reflected by the statistics on occupational accidents (Smolander, Louhevaaral, & Oja, 1984).

However, administrators in many of the country's police and fire departments are grappling with the problems of on-duty injury and off duty illness by instituting fitness and conditioning programs for their personnel, often cooperation with exercise physiologists and sports medicine centers (Mealey, 1979).

1.2 Yoga

Yoga is a group of physical, mental, and spiritual practices or disciplines which originated in ancient India. Yoga is one of the 6th orthodox schools of Hindu philosophical traditions (Feuerstein, 1998). The great sage Patanjali who was born in 200 BC systematic the science of yoga which was being handed down by word of mouth from one generation to another. Traditionally it said that Lord Siva was the innovator of yoga. Yoga is explained vividly in the great scriptures like Vedas, Upanishads, Gita and Ramayana (Gnanabakthan, 2011).

Classical Yoga or Astanga Yoga (Yoga of eight limbs) is mainly the type of Yoga such as Yama, Niyama, Asana, Pranayama, Pratyahara, dharana, Dhyana and Samadhi outlined in the highly influential (Yoga Sutras of Patanjali, White, David Gordon, 2014)

1.3 Yoga for Policeman

Yoga could come from the outside appear as just a physical exercise to tone the body, but its benefits lies buried only to be unraveled with persistent practice. The Police officials have turned to Yoga, to beat their work stress due to their excited lifestyle. Yoga Asanas apart from contributing to the physical fitness of and human being extends to calm and sooth the mind paving way for deeper relaxation for stress management. This in turn helps for more increased productivity in one's career, here with the police department, to curb crime (Gnanabakthan, 2011).

1.4 Integrated Yoga module

The basis of developing the integrated approach is ancient *Yoga* texts for total physical, mental, emotional, social, and spiritual levels development (Lokeswarananda, & Taittiriya, 1996; Nagarathna, & Nagendra, 2003). The techniques include physical practices (Kriyās, Āsanās, a healthy Yogic diet), breathing practices with body movements and Pranayama, meditation, lectures on Yoga, stress management, and life-style change through notional corrections for blissful awareness under all circumstances (action in relaxation) (Amaranath, Nagendra, & Deshpande, 2016).

1.4.1 Asana

The practice of physical posture is called as asana. It is most normally known aspect of yoga for those unfamiliar with the other 7 limbs. The verbal meaning of asana is staying or abiding asana is one way in which a person can experience the unity of body and mind (Moghe, 2015).

Asana is defined as which is comfortable and easy as well as firm. Asana are prescribed for the purpose of comfort during meditation and the practice of pranayama. Asana is dynamic position in which the practitioner is perfectly poised between activities and non-activity. Patanjali stated that asana and pranayama practices will bring about the desired state of health: the control of breath and our attention upon a single object, sensation, utterance, issue, mental state or activity (Naranjo, & Ornstein, 1971).

While the concentration on meditation involves focusing attention on one object, the mindfulness meditation aims at focusing attention on the field. In both the practices, the procedure involves 'retraining' of attention. He pointed out while describing meditation that "the need for the mediator to retrain his attention, whether through concentration or mindfulness, is the single invariant ingredient in the recipe for altering consciousness of every meditation system (Rao, 1989).

1.4.2 Kriyas

Yogic kriya or shat (six) - kriyas, it has been explained in Niyama of eight limbs of yoga that one has to do the practice of yogic kriya cleaning techniques. Used to purify the body and mind which ultimately open the pathways of nadis in the body and the energy in the body, in the mind and in the heart. Kriya more popularly called shat (six) kriyas. They are six in number commonly known as Dhauti, Bhasti, Neti, Trataka, Nauli and Kapalbhati (Moghe, 2015).

1.5 Benefits of yoga

Yoga simultaneously deals with all aspects of the philosophy, psychology and practicality of conscious evolution (Bhavanani, 2011). Yoga improved joint flexibility (US Ray, Purkayastha, Asnani, Tomer, Prashad, Thakur, & Selvamurthy, 2001), respiratory endurance, and strengthening of muscles (Nambinarayanan, Thakur, Krishnamurthy, & Chandrabose, 1992). The other documented physical health benefits of Yoga are reduction in body fat, improved in shoulder flexibility (Chen, & Tseng, 2008) improvement in immunological tolerance (Solberg, Halvorsen, Sundgot-Borgen, Ingjer, & Holen, 1995). The utility of yoga in improving mood and the differential effects may be related to its influence on physiological states of arousal (West, Otte, Geher, Johnson, & Mohr, 2004).

1.6 Reasons for the Selection of Topic

Health is the chief wealth for any human being. Only a healthy body would lead to a healthy mind. Police personnel with extended working hours and untimely food habits were vulnerable for stress and ailments. In the absence of good health, family and work would suffer, he added.

In this study, the researcher was interested to highlight the effect of integrated yoga modules on selected physical fitness variables, physiological and psychological variables of Policemen.

The researcher made an attempt a study on this area due to the lack of literature and studies in the same fields, and especially Police men. Hence, the researcher wants to find out the effect of yogic practice separately among Police men.

1.7 Statement of the Problem

Keeping the above aspects, the purpose of the study was to find out the effect of integrated yoga modules on selected physical fitness, physiological and psychological variables among Police men.

Particularly, the study was planned to examine if there were any significant differences in physical fitness (cardio vascular endurance and muscular endurance), physiological (resting pulse rate, and breathe holding time) and psychological (stress and self-confidence) parameters among Police men due to the effect of integrated Yoga Modules from the baseline measures to the post tests.

1.8 Research Questions

In this study, the following research questions were used to reveal if the effect of integrated Yoga modules training make any changes on selected Physical fitness, Physiological and Psychological variables among Police men.

Would the 12 week integrated Yoga module programme improve the physical fitness variable in the presence of covariate (control)?

Would the 12 week integrated Yoga module programme improve the physiological variables in the presence of covariate (control)?

Would the 12 week integrated Yoga module programme improve the psychological variables in the presence of covariate (control)?

Would the experimental group differ with control group in improving the physical fitness, physiological and psychological variables among Police men?

1.9 Assumptions

The validity of this study will rely on the following assumptions:

1. Subjects were adhered the integrated yoga module training protocol correctly.

2. Subjects performed the assigned training sessions for three days per week.

3. Subjects did not undergo any vigorous exercise during the course experimental period.

4. Subjects were tested accurately by using standardized test items to assess the selected dependent variables.

5. Subjects compiled with the best of their ability to the training and testing directions.

1.10 Delimitations

The study was delimited in the following factors.

1. To achieve the purpose of the study, 30 Police men were selected at random as subjects from Tamil Nadu Special Police 9th and 12th Battalion, Manimuthar, Tirunelveli district, Tamil Nadu, India.

2. The age of the subjects ranged from 26 and 34 years.

3. The selected subject were divided into two groups, namely such as experimental (n=15) and control (n=15) groups.

4. The duration of training was restricted for a period of 12 weeks and the number of sessions per week was confined to three.

5. Each training session was held for 60-90 minutes, three days per week .

6. The study was delimited to the following dependent variables such as;

Physical Fitness

Cardio Vascular Endurance

Muscular Endurance

Physiological Variables

Resting Pulse Rate

Breath Holding Time

Psychological variables

Stress

Self-confidence

7. The data on pre and posttests were collected on all the selected dependent variables two days prior and immediately after the intervention period respectively.

8. Training sessions would be conducted and supervised by the researcher.

1.11 Limitations

The following limitations were not considered while interpreting the findings of the present study.

1. Psychological factors, food habits, rest period and life style could not be controlled.

2. The weather conditions such as atmospheric temperature, humidity and meteorological factors during testing period were also not considered

3. Though the subjects were motivated verbally, no attempt was made to differentiate the motivation level during the period testing.

4. There are confounding variables which will not be controlled for: level of extracurricular activity and early intervention or lack of which may affect development of core control; confounding variables that the study will attempt to control by matching groups include: age, gender, height, weight

5. The sample is one of convenience in a suburban Tamil Nadu Special Police 9th and 12th Battalion, Manimuthar, Tirunelveli District. The area attracts cultural diversity, but it located in a socioeconomically affluent area.

6. We were unable to determine whether police had additional skill practice outside of home. However, verbal interactions with the police, and teacher report of sociality discussions suggested that police had little or no opportunity to be active at home.

1.12 Hypotheses

It has been scientifically accepted that any systematic training over a continuous period of time would lead to produce changes in the selected dependent variables. Based on the study, Conducted and reviewing the related literature available in the area, the investigator framed the following hypotheses and it was tested at 0.05 level of confidence.

First Hypothesis

H_0: It was hypothesized that the experimental group would not show significant improvement on selected physical fitness variables as a result of the 12 week integrated yoga module programme.

Ha: It was hypothesized that the experimental group would show significant improvement on Physical fitness variables as a result of the 12 week integrated yoga module programme.

Second Hypothesis

H_0: It was hypothesized that the Experimental group would not show significant improvement on selected physiological variables as a result of the 12 week integrated yoga module programme.

Ha: It was hypothesized that the Experimental group would show significant improvement on selected physiological variables as a result of the 12 week integrated yoga module programme.

Third Hypothesis

H_0: It was hypothesized that the Experimental group would not show significant improvement on selected psychological variables as a result of the 12 week integrated yoga module programme.

Ha: It was hypothesized that the Experimental group would show significant improvement on selected psychological variables as a result of the 12 week integrated yoga module programme.

Fourth Hypothesis

H_0: It was hypothesized that the control group would not show significant improvement between pre and posttests on selected physical fitness, Physiological and psychological variables.

Ha: It was hypothesized that the control group would show significant improvement between pre and posttests on selected physical fitness, Physiological and psychological variables.

Fifth Hypothesis

H_0: It was also hypothesized that the experimental group had not shown significant difference on selected physical fitness, physiological and psychological variables when compared with control group.

H_a: It was also hypothesized that the experimental group had shown significant difference on selected physical fitness, physiological and psychological variables when compared with control group.

1.13 Significance of the Study

The results of the study may contribute in the following ways;

1. The findings of the study would explore the status of the integrated yoga module among Police men.

2. The findings of the study will helpful for the further research studies, also helpful for the academy of among Police men.

3. This study would give an exact idea about physical fitness variables like how to develop the cardio vascular endurance and muscular endurance.

4. This study would give an exact idea about physiological variables like decrease of resting pulse rate and breathe holding time.

5. This study would give an exact idea about psychological variables like reducing stress and improve the self-confidence level.

1.14 Definition of the Operational Terms

1.14.1 Yoga

The literal meaning of the Sanskrit word Yoga is 'Yoke'. Yoga can therefore be defined as a means of uniting the individual spirit with the universal spirit of God. According to Maharishi Patanjali, Yoga is the suppression of modifications of the mind.

1.14.2 Integrated Yoga Module

Integrated Yoga module (IYM) consisting of physical postures (Asana), voluntary regulation of breathing (Pranayama), maintaining silence and visual focusing exercises (Trataka) (Telles, Hanumanthaiah, Nagarathna, & Nagendra, 1993).

1.14.3 Cardio vascular endurance

Cardiovascular fitness is the ability of the heart and lungs to supply oxygen-rich blood to the working muscle tissues, and the ability of the muscles to use oxygen to produce energy for movement (National Physical Activity Guidelines).

1.14.4 Muscular endurance

Baumgartner, & Jackson, (1991) defined muscular endurance as "The ability of a muscle or group of muscles to overcome resistance or to act against resistance for longer duration under conditions of fatigue or tiredness

1.14.5 Resting heart rate

The number of pulse beats per unit time, usually per minute. The pulse rate is based on the number of contractions of the ventricles (the lower chambers of the heart). The pulse rate may be too fast (tachycardia) or too slow (bradycardia) (Karvonen, 1957).

1.14.6 Breath holding time

Breath holding time is defined as the duration of time through which one can hold his breathe without the study of all living things (Morehouse, & Miller, 1967).

1.14.7 Stress

Stress may be defined as the "Response pattern of an organism to prepare itself for Fight or Flight (Walter, 1932).

1.14.8 Self-confidence

The concept of self-confidence is commonly used as self-assurance in one's personal judgment, ability, power, etc. One's self confidence increases from experiences of having mastered particular activities (Snyder, & Lopez, (Eds.) 2009).

1.15 Organization of the Dissertation.

This dissertation includes five chapters. The first chapter is an introductory chapter that provides a brief explanation of the sports training, purposes of the study, boundaries of the study, generation of research hypotheses and significance of the study.

The second chapter is the literature review. It introduces information about the dependent and independent variables, and describes the theoretical under the effects of independent variable on dependent variables.

The third chapter describes research methodology. It consists of training and testing procedures, measures, sample selection, and data analysis procedures.

In the fourth chapter, analysis of the collected data was presented. It includes results of measurement and structural model tests, and hypotheses tests.

The fifth chapter discusses the findings and conclusions of the research, as well as implications and recommendations for future research.

Chapter II

REVIEW OF RELATED LITERATURE

2.1 Introduction

A study of relevant literature is an essential step to get a full picture of what has been done with regard to the problem under the study. Such a review brings new ideas, theories, comparative materials and helps in the development of research procedure. The research scholar had come across general books, periodicals, journals, internet and unpublished theses while searching for relevant facts and findings that are related to the present study. Such of these facts are given below for a better understanding and to justify this study.

The phrase "review of literature" consists of two words "review" and "literature". In research methodology, the term literature refers to the knowledge of a particular area of any discipline which includes theoretical practical and its research studies.

The literature in any field forms the foundation upon which the future work will be built. If we fail to build foundation of knowledge provided by the review of literature one work is likely to be shadow and that has already done better by someone else.

The following review of literature addresses the effect of integrated yoga module training on physical fitness, physiological and psychological parameters. Terms relevant to the study in this thesis are operationally defined. The literature in any field forms the foundation upon which all future work will be built. If we fail to build upon the foundation of knowledge provided by the review of literature, the researcher might miss some works already done on the same topic.

2.2 Studies on integrated Yoga Module

Satyapriya, Nagendra., Nagarathna, & Padmalatha (2009) studied the effect of integrated yoga practice and guided yogic relaxation on both perceived stress and measured autonomic response in healthy pregnant women. The 122 healthy women recruited between the 18th and 20th week of pregnancy at prenatal clinics in Bangalore, India, were randomized to practicing yoga and deep relaxation or standard prenatal exercises 1hour daily. The results for the 45 participants per group who completed the study were evaluated by repeated measures analysis of variance. Yoga reduces perceived stress and improves adaptive autonomic response to stress in healthy pregnant women.

Rakhshani, Maharana, Raghuram, Nagendra, & Venkatram (2010) investigated the effects of integrated yoga on the quality of life and interpersonal relationships in normal pregnant women. One hundred and two pregnant women between 18 and 20 weeks of gestation who met the inclusion criteria were recruited from the obstetric units in Bangalore and were randomly assigned to two groups of yoga (n = 51) and control (n = 51). Women with medical conditions that could potentially lead to pregnancy complications and those with abnormal fetal parameters were excluded. The yoga group received integrated yoga while control group received standard antenatal exercises, both for 1-h three times a week from 20th to 36th week of gestation. Pre and post assessments were done using WHOQOL-100 and FIRO-B questionnaires. The integrated yoga is an efficacious means of improving the quality of life of pregnant women and enhancing certain aspects of their interpersonal relationships.

Ganpat, Nagendra (2011) assessed mental health in managers undergoing yoga-based Self-Management of Excessive Tension (SMET) program.72 managers with 48.75±3.86 years of mean age were participated in this study of single group pre-post design. The General Health Questionnaire data were taken on the first and sixth day of 5 days SMET programThese results suggest that participation in a SMET program was associated with improvement in mental health and may have implications for "Executive Efficiency."

Narasimhan, Nagarathna, & Nagendra (2011) examined the safety and feasibility of conducting a weeklong free yoga camp, and (ii) assess its impact on the negative and positive affect in normal healthy volunteers.In this open-arm study450 participants were taught integrated yoga module. It included asanas, pranayama, relaxation, notional correction and devotional sessions. Assessment was carried out on the first and last day of the camp, using a modified version of Positive Affect Negative Affect Scale (PANAS). It has ten questions each to measure positive (PA) and negative affect (NA). Nine questions have been added which are referred as other positive affect (OPA) and other negative affect (ONA) domains.It is feasible and safe to conduct a weeklong yoga camp in an urban setting, and integrated yoga practices can reduce the negative affect and increase the positive affect within one week.

Ram, Raghuram, Rao, Bhargav, Koka, Tripathi, Nelamangala, Kodaganur, Ramarao (2012) presented the theoretical basis and validate the need based holistic yoga modules for cancer patients. Literature from traditional texts including Vedas, Ayurveda, Upanishads, Bhagavat Gita, Yoga Vasishtha etc. and their commentaries were looked into for references of cancer and therapeutic directives. Present day scientific literature was also explored with regards to defining cancer, its etiopathology and its management. Results of studies done using CAM therapies were also looked at, for salient findings. Focused group discussions (FGD) amongst researchers, experienced gurus, and medical professionals involved in research and clinical cancer practice were carried out with the objectives of determining needs of the patient and yoga practices that could prove efficient. A list of needs at different stages of conventional therapies (surgery, chemotherapy and radiation therapy) was listed and yoga modules were developed accordingly. Considering the needs, expected side effects, the energy levels and the psychological states of the participants, eight modules evolved. The evidence from the traditional knowledge and recent scientific studies validates eight modules of the integrated approach of yoga therapy for cancer that can be used safely and effectively as complimentary during all conventional cancer therapies.

Ebnezar, Nagarathna, Yogitha, & Nagendra (2012) studied the effect of integrated yoga on pain, morning stiffness and anxiety in osteoarthritis of knees. Two hundred and fifty participants with OA knees (35–80 years) were randomly assigned to yoga or control group. Both groups had transcutaneous electrical stimulation and ultrasound treatment followed by intervention (40 min) for two weeks with follow up for three months. The integrated yoga consisted of yogic loosening and strengthening practices, *asanas*, relaxation, *pranayama* and meditation. The control group had physiotherapy exercises. Assessments were done on 15th (post 1) and 90th day (post 2). Integrated approach of yoga therapy is better than physiotherapy exercises as an adjunct to transcutaneous electrical stimulation and ultrasound treatment in reducing pain, morning stiffness, state and trait anxiety, blood pressure and pulse rate in patients with OA knees.

Naveen, Rao, Vishal, Thirthalli, Varambally, Gangadhar (2013) developed a comprehensive yoga therapy module targeting specific clinical features of depression. Specific yoga practices were matched for clinical features of depression based on a thorough literature review. A yoga program was developed, which consisted of Sukṣmavyayāma, (loosening exercises), äsanas (postures), relaxation techniques, Pranayama (breathing exercises) and chanting meditation to be taught in a 2 week period. A structured questionnaire was developed for validation from nine experienced yoga professionals. The final version of yoga therapy module was pilot-tested on seven patients (five females) with depression recruited from The developed comprehensive yoga therapy module was validated by experts in the field and was found to be feasible and useful in patients with depression.

Satyapriya, Nagarathna, Padmalatha, & Nagendra (2013) studied the effect of integrated yoga on Pregnancy experience, anxiety, and depression in normal pregnancy. This Prospective Randomized control study recruited 96 women in 20th week of normal pregnancy. Yoga group ($n = 51$) practiced integrated yoga and control group ($n = 45$) did standard antenatal exercises, one hour daily, from 20th to 36th week of gestation. Mann–Whitney and Wilcoxon's tests were used for statistical analysis. Yoga reduces anxiety, depression and pregnancy related uncomfortable experiences.

Maharana, Nagarathna, Padmalatha, Nagendra, & Hankey (2013) investigated the effect of yoga on labor outcome. This randomized two-armed active control study recruited 96 women with normal pregnancy. The experimental group practiced integrated yoga and the control group practiced standard antenatal exercises (1 hr/day), from 18 to 20 weeks of gestation until term. Yoga during pregnancy decreases the duration of all stages of labor, complications of pregnancy, need for epidural analgesia, and cesarean sections. it also improves birth weight and Apgar scores of the infant.

Parthasarathy, Jaiganesh, & Duraisamy (2014) compared the effects of asanas, yoga as an integrated module, on selected psychological variables among women with anxiety problem. The sample for the present study consists of 45 women with anxiety disorder from a tertiary care centre at Chennai city near Puducherry. After proper institutional ethics committee approval, the subjects were selected using random sampling method. Their ages ranged from 25 to 35 years. They were divided into three groups by a sealed envelope technique, namely Experimental group I, Experimental group II and Control group (III). Experimental group I was administered asanas, pranayamas and relaxation for a period of eight weeks in the morning and Experimental group II was under the practice of Sitilikarana vyayama, suryanamaskar, asanas, pranayama and yoga nidra practices (integrated yoga module) for a period of eight weeks. The training programme was administered for forty-five minutes per session. The control group did not engage in any special activities. The described yogic practices were done according to established protocols. The detailed description of the techniques is beyond the scope of this article. The load of the treatment was based on a pilot study. Anxiety was measured by Taylor's Manifest Anxiety Scale before and after treatment. Frustration was measured through Reaction to Frustration Scale. All data were spread in an Excel sheet to be analysed with SPSS 16 software using analysis of covariance (ANCOVA). The practice of asanas, relaxation and pranayama decreased anxiety in women but the practice of yoga as an integrated yoga module significantly improved anxiety scores in young women with proven anxiety without any ill effects.

Patil, (2014) developed and standardize an inventory to assess the prakrti and understand the effect of Integral Yoga Module on the tridoshas and trigunas in children.The parent rating scales Ayurveda Child Personality inventory, Ayurveda Guna inventory for children and Self-rating scales Caraka Child Personality Inventory, Sushruta Child Personality Inventory were developed on the basis of translation of Sanskrit verses describing Vātaja (A), Pittaja (B). Kapha (C)., Sattva (A), Rajas(B) and Tamas prakrti (C) characteristics and by taking the opinions of Ayurveda experts and psychologists. The scales was tested out in Maxwell public school and New Generation National Public School, to Bangalore. The scale was administered on children of the age group 6-12 and 8-12 years. There were two studies involved. One was design and other was pre-post design with control. For randomized-control study 100 children from New Generation National public school, were randomly assigned to Yoga and control group. And for Personality camp study , 320 children(160 children in each group), aged 8-12 yrs, selected from a residential camp at Prashanti kutiram Jigani (experimental group) and Jayagopal Garodia Rasrtothana school. Experimental group children practiced Integral Yoga module including Asanas, pranayama, nadanusandhana, 5 chanting, and games. Control group children observed were not given any intervention. Caraka Child personality inventory and Sushruta Child Personality Inventory were administered before and after one month (RCT study), 10 days (PDC study). Mann Whitney U test and Wilcoxon Signed Ranks Test were applied. The prakrti (tridoshas and trigunas) of the children can be measured reliably by Ayurveda Child Personality inventory, Ayurveda guna inventory for children and Caraka Child Personality Inventory, Sushruta Child Personality Inventory. Correlation with parent rating scale suggested criterion –related validity. Integral Yoga module has the significant effect on the tridoshas (Vata,Pitta and Kapha) and trigunas (Sattva, Rajas and Tamas) in Children.

Rao, Raghuram, Nagendra, Usharani, Gopinath, Diwakar, Patil, Bilimagga, (2015) compared the effects of yoga program with supportive therapy on self-reported symptoms of depression in breast cancer patients undergoing conventional treatment. Ninety-eight breast cancer patients with stage II and III disease from a cancer center were randomly assigned to receive yoga (n = 45) and supportive therapy (n = 53) over a 24-week period during which they underwent surgery followed by adjuvant radiotherapy (RT) or chemotherapy (CT) or both. The study stoppage criteria was progressive disease rendering the patient bedridden or any physical musculoskeletal injury resulting from intervention or less than 60% attendance to yoga intervention. Subjects underwent yoga intervention for 60 min daily with control group undergoing supportive therapy during their hospital visits. Beck's Depression Inventory (BDI) and symptom checklist were assessed at baseline, after surgery, before, during, and after RT and six cycles of CT. We used analysis of covariance (intent-to-treat) to study the effects of intervention on depression scores and Pearson correlation analyses to evaluate the bivariate relationships. The results suggest possible antidepressant effects with yoga intervention in breast cancer patients undergoing conventional treatment.

Patil, Nagarathna, Tekur, Patil, Nagendra, Subramanya (2015) reported the development, validation, and feasibility of an integrated yoga therapy module (IYTM) for CLBP. In the first phase, IYTM for CLBP was designed based on the literature review of classical texts and recently published research studies. In the second phase, designed IYTM (26 yoga practices) was validated by thirty subject matter (yoga) experts. Content validity ratio (CVR) was analyzed using Lawshe's formula. In the third phase, the validated IYTM (20 yoga practices) was tested on 12 patients for pain, disability and perceived stress at baseline and after 1-month of this intervention. The designed IYTM was validated by thirty yoga experts and later evaluated on a small sample. This study has shown that the validated IYTM is feasible, had no adverse effects and was useful in alleviating pain, disability, and perceived stress in patients with CLBP. However, randomized control trials with larger sample are needed to strengthen the study.

Patil, Nagarathna, Tekur, Patil, Nagendra, & Subramanya (2015) carried out a study at the SVYASA Yoga University, Bengaluru, South India. The IYTM for CLBP was designed, validated, and later tested for feasibility in patients with CLBP. In the first phase, IYTM for CLBP was designed based on the literature review of classical texts and recently published research studies. In the second phase, designed IYTM (26 yoga practices) was validated by thirty subject matter (yoga) experts. Content validity ratio (CVR) was analyzed by using Lawshe's formula. In the third phase, the validated IYTM (20 yoga practices) was tested on 12 patients for pain, disability and perceived stress at baseline and after 1-month of this intervention. The designed IYTM was validated by thirty yoga experts and later evaluated on a small sample. This study has shown that the validated IYTM is feasible, had no adverse effects and was useful in alleviating pain, disability, and perceived stress in patients with CLBP. However, randomized control trials with larger sample are needed to strengthen the study.

Amaranath, (2015) To study the efficacy of Integrated Yoga Module (IYM) on Personality (Gunas) (Yogic personality measure) of HGs, on Emotions (Positive and Negative Affect) of Home Guards (HGs), on Perceived stress and Satisfaction with life of HG's and on Verbal Aggression of HG's. Subjects were selected from 500 HGs working on field, from Bangalore Rural District who attended motivational lectures presented by the competent instructors. 148 HGs, volunteered to take part in the study were randomly divided into YG (n=75) and CG (n=73) using a Random number calculator [Internet], random number table was generated Of the 75 subjects in YG and 73 subjects in CG, the age ranged between 20 and 50 years. There was 36 and 31 female in YG and CG respectively, similarly there was 39 and 42 male in YG and CG category. 49 were married both in YG and CG, 26 in YG and 24 in unmarried. Educational qualifications ranged from Non-matriculate to graduate. This is a randomized controlled prospective study of normal HGs assessing efficacy of an IYM for eight weeks on148 normal adults to change their personality (Guna) as assessed by VPI. Results have shown that there is an increase in Sattva level (P) < 0.001 in YG and decrease in CG. There was significant decreases in Rajas and Tamas in YG and increases in CG. When data analysis was subdivided by gender, educational qualification and age all categories showed similar trends as expected according to the Yogic literature. There was an increase in Sattva in Yoga group whereas it has decreased in controlled group. Rajas and Tamas significantly decreased in Yoga group whereas it has increased in controlled group. Hence, integrated Yoga module can be suggested for Home Guards which are cost effective and helps them for coping up with stressful situations. The improvement observed in Yoga group, after eight weeks of intervention in all variables, has shown that Yoga could be an equally effective and cost effective tool. It also points out the utility of the VPI as a tool for measuring the subtle dimensions of Guna described in traditional texts of Yoga that can measure the steps of growth of an individual.

Nagendra, (2015) studied the efficacy of Integrated Yoga Module (IYM) on PSS, VAS and SWL in HGs. Five HGs who attended introductory lectures, 148 HGs of both sexes, who satisfied the inclusion and exclusion criteria were randomly allocated into two groups. The *Yoga* group (YG) practiced in an IYM that included Asanas, Pranayama, meditation and lectures. The control group (CG) was not given any *Yoga* practice but they were performing their routine work. The experimental group had supervised practice sessions for one hour daily, six days a week for eight weeks. Perceived Stress, Verbal Aggression and Satisfaction in Life was assessed before and after 8 weeks using the self-administered PSS, VAS and SWL Scale. There was a significant decrease in PSS, VAS level in the *YG* and a significant increase in the CG. PSS, VAS was also found significant in between groups, similarly there was a significant increase in SWL level in *YG* with a significant decrease in the CG. SWL was also found significant in between groups. This study has showed that 8 week intervention of IYM reduced Perceived Stress Level, Verbal aggression in the *YG* and it increased in the CG. Also Satisfaction in Life level increased in *YG* and decreased in CG.

Rshikesan, & Subramanya (2016) assessed the effect of Integrated Approach of Yoga Therapy (IAYT) yoga module on adult male obesity in an urban setting. RCT (Randomized Controlled Trial) was conducted for 14 weeks on obese male subjects with yoga and control groups. Total number of subjects were 72 and they were randomized into two groups (Yoga n=37, Control n=35). The subjects are from an urban setting of Mumbai and are from doing yoga for the first time. Special yoga training of IAYT was given to yoga group for one and half an hour for 5 days in a week for 14 weeks. The control group continued regular physical activities and no specific physical activity was given. The assessments were anthropometric parameters of weight, Body Mass Index (BMI), MAC (Mid Upper Arm Circumferences) of Left and Right Arm, Waist Circumference (WC), HC (Hip Circumference), WHR (Waist Hip Ratio), SKF (Skin Fold Thickness of Biceps, Triceps, Sub scapular, suprailiac and cumulative), Percentage body fat based on SKF and Psychological Questionnaires of Perceived Stress Scale (PSS) and AAQW (Acceptance and Action Questionnaire for Weight Related Difficulty). These are taken before and after intervention for both yoga and control groups. Within and between group analysis & correlation of differences from post to pre readings among the variables, were carried out using SPSS 21.Incorporating the IAYT for obese male in urban setting will be effective for obesity treatment and for reducing the obesity related problems.

Amaranath, Nagendra, & Deshpande (2016) studied the efficacy of integrated *Yoga* module (IYM) on emotions (positive and negative affect [PA and NA]) of HGs A total of 148 HGs both males and females who qualified the inclusion and exclusion criteria were randomly divided into *Yoga* group (YG) and control groups (CG). The YG had supervised practice sessions (by trained experts) for 1 h daily, 6 days a week for 8 weeks along with their regular routine work whereas CG performing their routine work. Positive affect negative affect scale (PANAS) was assessed before and after 8 weeks using a modified version of PANAS. The results suggested that IYM can be useful for HGs to improve the PA and to decrease NA score. Moreover, IYM is cost-effective and helps HGs for coping up with emotions in stressful situations.

Chobe, Bhargav, Raghuram, & Garner (2016) assessed the effect of integrated Yoga and Physical therapy (IYP) on audiovisual reaction times, depression and anxiety in patients suffering from chronic MS. From a neuro-rehabilitation center in Germany, 11 patients (six females) suffering from MS for 19 ± 7.4 years were recruited. Subjects were in the age range of 55.45 ± 10.02 years and had Extended Disability Status Scores (EDSS) below 7. All the subjects received mind–body intervention of integrated Yoga and Physical therapy (IYP) for 3 weeks. The intervention was given in a residential setup. Patients followed a routine involving Yogic physical postures, pranayama, and meditations along with various Physical therapy (PT) techniques for 21 days, 5 days a week, 5 h/day. They were assessed before and after intervention for changes in audiovisual reaction times (using Brain Fit Model No. OT 400), anxiety, and depression [using Hospital Anxiety and Depression Scale (HADS)]. Data was analyzed using paired samples test. This pilot project suggests utility of IYP intervention for improving audiovisual reaction times and psychological health in chronic MS patients. In future, randomized controlled trials with larger sample size should be performed to confirm these findings.

Naoroibam, Metri, Bhargav, Nagaratna, & Nagendra (2016) studied the effect of 1-month integrated yoga (IY) intervention on anxiety, depression, and CD4 counts in patients suffering from HIV-1 infection. Forty four HIV-1 infected individuals from two HIV rehabilitation centers of Manipur State of India were randomized into two groups: Yoga ($n = 22$; 12 males) and control ($n = 22$; 14 males). Yoga group received IY intervention, which included physical postures (asanas), breathing practices (pranayama), relaxation techniques, and meditation. IY sessions were given 60 min/day, 6 days a week for 1 month. Control group followed daily routine during this period. All patients were on anti-retroviral therapy (ART) and dosages were kept stable during the study. There was no significant difference in age, gender, education, CD4 counts, and ART status between the two groups. Hospital anxiety and depression scale was used to assess anxiety and depression, CD4 counts were measured by flow cytometry before and after intervention. Analysis of variance – repeated measures was applied to analyze the data using SPSS version 10.One month practice of IY may reduce depression and improve immunity in HIV-1 infected adults.

Chobe, Bhargav, Raghuram, Garner (2016) assessed the effect of integrated Yoga and Physical therapy (IYP) on audiovisual reaction times, depression and anxiety in patients suffering from chronic MS. From a neuro-rehabilitation center in Germany, 11 patients (six females) suffering from MS for 19 ± 7.4 years were recruited. Subjects were in the age range of 55.45 ± 10.02 years and had Extended Disability Status Scores (EDSS) below 7. All the subjects received mind-body intervention of integrated Yoga and Physical therapy (IYP) for 3 weeks. The intervention was given in a residential setup. Patients followed a routine involving Yogic physical postures, pranayama, and meditations along with various Physical therapy (PT) techniques for 21 days, 5 days a week, 5 h/day. They was assessed before and after intervention for changes in audiovisual reaction times (using Brain Fit Model No. OT 400), anxiety, and depression [using Hospital Anxiety and Depression Scale (HADS)]. Data was analyzed by using paired samples test. This pilot project suggests utility of IYP intervention for improving audiovisual reaction times and psychological health in chronic MS patients. In future, randomized controlled trials with larger sample size should be performed to confirm these findings.

Amaranath , Nagendra , Deshpande (2016) studied the efficacy of integrated yoga module (IYM) on personality (Gunās) (yogic personality measure) of HGs. Of 500 HGs who attended introductory lectures, 148 HGs of either gender, who satisfied the inclusion and exclusion criteria and who consented to participate in the study were randomly allocated for two groups. The yoga group (YG) practiced an IYM for 1 h daily, 6 days a week for 8 weeks along with their routine work. The control group (CG) remained on routine work. Personality was assessed before and after 8 weeks using the self-administered Vedic Personality Inventory. Indicate that IYM can profitably be suggested for HGs as a cost-effective means to help them cope with stressful situations.

Kakde, Metri, Varambally, Nagaratna, & Nagendra, (2017) developed and validated an integrated yoga module(IYM) for PD. The IYM was prepared after a thorough review of classical yoga texts and previous findings. Twenty experienced yoga experts, who fulfilled the inclusion criteria, were selected validating the content of the IYM. A total of 28 practices were included in the IYM, and each practice was discussed and rated as (i) not essential, (ii) useful but not essential, and (iii) essential; the content validity ratio (CVR) was calculated using Lawshe's formula. The IYM is valid for PD, with good content validity. However, future studies must determine the feasibility and efficacy of the developed module

Pise Pradhan, & Gharote (2017) aimed at developing a validated YM for children with IDs. The content validity of YM for children with IDs was assessed by a panel of 22 experienced yoga experts. The YM for children with IDs was developed in the form of tailor-made yoga practices that were supported by classical texts and research evidence. A total of 32 practices were included in the YM, and each practice was discussed and rated as (i) not essential, (ii) useful but not essential, and (iii) essential. The content validity ratio was calculated using Lawshe's formula. The present study suggests that the YM for children with IDs is valid with good content validity. However, future randomized controlled trials must determine the feasibility and efficacy of the developed YM for children with IDs.

Verma, Bhargav, Varambally, Raghuram, & Gangadhar (2018) discussed with Twenty one (12 females) subjects, diagnosed with schizophrenia by a psychiatrist using ICD-10, in the ages $52.87 + 9.5$ years and suffering since 24.0 ± 3.05 years were recruited into the study from a schizophrenia rehabilitation center in Bengaluru. All subjects were taking anti-psychotic medications and were in stable state for more than a month. Psychiatric medications were kept constant during the study period. Assessments were done at three points of time: (1) baseline, (2) after one month of usual routine (pre) and (3) after five months of validated Integrated Yoga (IY) intervention (post). Validated 1 h Yoga module (consisting of asanas, pranayama, relaxation techniques and chantings) was practiced for 5 months, five sessions per week. Antipsychotic-induced side effects were assessed using Simpson Angus Scale (SAS) and Udvalg for Kliniske Undersogelser (UKU) side effect rating scale. Cognitive functions (using Trail making Test A and B), clinical symptoms and anthropometry were assessed as secondary variables. Comparisons between "pre" and "post" data was done using paired samples t-tests after subtracting baseline scores from them respectively. The present study provides preliminary evidence for usefulness of Integrated Yoga intervention in managing anti-psychotic-induced side effects.

Balakrishnan, Nanjundaiah, Nirwan, Sharma, Ganju, Saha, & Ramarao (2019) examined the Yoga module for better management of stressors in extreme environmental condition of Antarctica. A Yoga module was designed based on the traditional and contemporary yoga literature as well as published studies. The Yoga module was sent for validation to forty experts of thirty responded. A specific yoga module for coping and facilitating adaptation in Antarctica was designed and validated. This module was used in the 35th Indian Scientific expedition to Antarctica, and experiments are underway to understand the efficacy and utility of Yoga on psychological stress, sleep, serum biomarkers and gene expression. Further outcomes shall provide the efficacy and utility of this module in Antarctic environments.

Balakrishnan Nanjundaiah, Nirwan, Sharma, Ganju Saha, Singh Ramarao (2019) described preparation of a Yoga module for better management of stressors in extreme environmental condition of Antarctica. A Yoga module was designed based on the traditional and contemporary yoga literature as well as published studies. The Yoga module was sent for validation to forty experts of which thirty responded .A specific yoga module for coping and facilitating adaptation in Antarctica was designed and validated. This module was used in the 35th Indian Scientific expedition to Antarctica, and experiments are underway to understand the efficacy and utility of Yoga on psychological stress, sleep, serum biomarkers and gene expression. Further outcomes shall provide the efficacy and utility of this module in Antarctic environments.

Naoroibam, Metri, Bhargav, Nagaratna, Nagendra (2016) studied the effect of 1-month integrated yoga (IY) intervention on anxiety, depression, and CD4 counts in patients suffering from HIV-1 infection. Forty four HIV-1 infected individuals from two HIV rehabilitation centers of Manipur State of India were randomized into two groups: Yoga (n = 22; 12 males) and control (n = 22; 14 males). Yoga group received IY intervention, which included physical postures (asanas), breathing practices (pranayama), relaxation techniques, and meditation. IY sessions were given 60 min/day, 6 days a week for 1 month. Control group followed daily routine during this period. All patients were on anti-retroviral therapy (ART) and dosages were kept stable during the study. There was no significant difference in age, gender, education, CD4 counts, and ART status between the two groups. Hospital anxiety and depression scale was used to assess anxiety and depression, CD4 counts were measured by flow cytometry before and after intervention. Analysis of variance - repeated measures was applied to analyze the data using SPSS version 10.One month practice of IY may reduce depression and improve immunity in HIV-1 infected adults.

Ebnezar, Nagarathna, Yogitha, Nagendra (2012) studied the effect of integrated yoga on pain, morning stiffness and anxiety in osteoarthritis of knees. Two hundred and fifty participants with OA knees (35-80 years) were randomly assigned to yoga or control group. Both groups had transcutaneous electrical stimulation and ultrasound treatment followed by intervention (40 min) for two weeks with follow up for three months. The integrated yoga consisted of yogic loosening and strengthening practices, asanas, relaxation, pranayama and meditation. The control group have physiotherapy exercises. Assessments were done on 15(th) (post 1) and 90(th) day (post 2).Integrated approach of yoga therapy is better than physiotherapy exercises as an adjunct to transcutaneous electrical stimulation and ultrasound treatment in reducing pain, morning stiffness, state and trait anxiety, blood pressure and pulse rate in patients with OA knees.

Nosaka, Okamura_(2012) conducted a case-control study with Ninety school employees. Three months after the intervention, the subjects were assigned to a daily practice group (case: n=43) and a nonconsecutive daily practice group (control: n=47) according to their daily practice level of the yoga therapy program. The subjects participated in a stress management education program based on an integrated yoga therapy session. The program included psychological education and counseling about stress management and yoga theories, as well as the practices of asanas, pranayama, relaxation, and cognitive structure based on Indian philosophy. Assessments were performed before and after the program using the Subjective Units of Distress for mind and body and the Two-Dimensional Mood Scale. The General Health Questionnaire 28 (GHQ28) was used to assess the mental health state before the intervention and at 3 months after the program. The present results suggested that a single session of an integrated yoga program was effective for reducing stress and that the mental health of school employees was promoted by the daily practice of the yoga therapy program.

Banerjee, Vadiraj, Ram, Rao, Jayapal, Gopinath, Ramesh, Rao, Kumar Raghuram, Hegde, Nagendra, Prakash Hande, (2007) studied the effects of an integrated yoga program in modulating perceived stress levels, anxiety, as well as depression levels and radiation-induced DNA damage in 68 breast cancer patients undergoing radiotherapy. Two psychological questionnaires--Hospital Anxiety and Depression Scale (HADS) and Perceived Stress Scale (PSS)--and DNA damage assay were used in the study. There was a significant decrease in the HADS scores in the yoga intervention group, whereas the control group displayed an increase in these scores. Mean PSS was decreased in the yoga group, whereas the control group did not show any change pre- and postradiotherapy. Radiation-induced DNA damage was significantly elevated in both the yoga and control groups after radiotherapy, but the postradiotherapy DNA damage in the yoga group was slightly less when compared to the control group. An integrated approach of yoga intervention modulates the stress and DNA damage levels in breast cancer patients during radiotherapy.

Raghavendra, Nagarathna, Nagendra, Gopinath, Srinath Ravi, Patil, Ramesh Nalini (2007) examined the effect of an integrated yoga programme on chemotherapy-related nausea and emesis in early operable breast cancer outpatients. Sixty-two subjects were randomly allocated to receive yoga (n = 28) or supportive therapy intervention (n = 34) during the course of their chemotherapy. Both groups have similar socio-demographic and medical characteristics. Intervention consist of both supervised and home practice of yoga sessions lasting for 60 min daily, while the control group received supportive therapy and coping preparation during their hospital visits over a complete course of chemotherapy. The primary outcome measure was the Morrow Assessment of Nausea and Emesis (MANE) assessed after the fourth cycle of chemotherapy. Secondary outcomes included measures for anxiety, depression, quality of life, distressful symptoms and treatment-related toxicity assessed before and during the course of chemotherapy. Following yoga, there was a significant decrease in post-chemotherapy-induced nausea frequency (P = 0.01) and nausea intensity (P = 0.01), and intensity of anticipatory nausea (P = 0.01) and anticipatory vomiting (P = 0.05) as compared with the control group. There was a significant positive correlation between MANE scores and anxiety, depression and distressful symptoms. In conclusion, the results suggest a possible use for stress reduction interventions such as yoga in complementing conventional antiemetics to manage chemotherapy-related nausea and emesis.

Rakhshani, Maharana, Raghuram, Nagendra, Venkatram (2016) investigated the effects of integrated yoga on the quality of life and interpersonal relationships in normal pregnant women. One hundred and two pregnant women between 18 and 20 weeks of gestation who met the inclusion criteria were recruited from the obstetric units in Bangalore and were randomly assigned to two groups of yoga (n = 51) and control (n = 51). Women with medical conditions that could potentially lead to pregnancy complications and those with abnormal fetal parameters were excluded. The yoga group received integrated yoga while control group received standard antenatal exercises, both for 1-h three times a week from 20th to 36th week of gestation. Pre and post assessments were done using WHOQOL-100 and FIRO-B questionnaires. The integrated yoga is an efficacious means of improving the quality of life of pregnant women and enhancing certain aspects of their interpersonal relationships.

Tolbaños Roche, Mas Hesse (2014) examined the efficacy of an integrative yoga programme as adjuvant treatment of essential arterial hypertension. An Integrative yoga programme was conducted during three months in 26 sessions with a group of ten essential arterial hypertension patients at a public health centre. The same number of patients acted as the control group without treatment. The patients were randomly selected and assigned to the groups. All patients filled in the Positive and Negative Affect Schedule (PANAS), the Hospital Anxiety and Depression Scale (HADS) and the Smith Relaxation States Inventory 3 (SRSI3) before and after the treatment. These positive and promising results confirm the effectiveness of these techniques in the treatment of essential arterial hypertension and suggest possible further investigations

Gopal, Mondal, Gandhi, Arora Bhattacharjee (2011) evaluated the impact of stress on psychological, physiological parameters, and immune system during medical term -academic examination and the effect of yoga practices on the same. The study was carried out on sixty first-year MBBS students randomly assigned to yoga group and control group (30 each). The yoga group underwent integrated yoga practices for 35 minutes daily in the presence of trained yoga teacher for 12 weeks. Control group did not undergo any kind of yoga practice or stress management. Physiological parameters like heart rate, respiratory rate, and blood pressure were measured. Global Assessment of Recent Stress Scale and Spielbergers State Anxiety score were assessed at baseline and during the examination. Serum cortisol levels, IL-4, and IFN-γ levels were determined by enzyme-linked immunosorbent assay technique. Yoga resists the autonomic changes and impairment of cellular immunity seen in examination stress.

According to Bhobe (2000) Yoga is a science of Holistic living and not merely a set of Asanas and Pranayama. It is a psycho physical and spiritual science, which aims at the harmonious development of the human body, mind and soul. Yoga is the conscious art of self-discovery. It is a process by which animal man ascends through the stages from normal man to super man and then the divine man. It is an expansion of the narrow constricted egoistic personality to an all-pervasive eternal and blissful state of reality. Yoga is an all-round development of personality at physical, mental intellectual, emotional and spiritual level.

Vinchurkar, Arankalle (2015) conducted a study with A 63-year-old overweight female prediagnosed of stress urinary incontinence presented with exacerbated events of urine leakage. She was advised a residential lifestyle and behavioral program, primarily consisting of a monitored yoga therapy module, apart from her ongoing anticholinergic medicine, for 21 days. Assessments were based on a frequency volume chart, a bladder diary for the entire duration of treatment, and the International Consultation on Incontinence Modular Questionnaire-Urinary Incontinence Short Form questionnaire on the days of admission and discharge. A total of 1.9 kg of weight loss was observed during her stay. Usage of pad, as reported in her diary, reduced from 3 to 1 per day. Her International Consultation on Incontinence Modular Questionnaire-Urinary Incontinence Short Form score reduced from 16 to 9, indicating better continence. She expressed subjective well-being and confidence in her social interactions. This is probably the first case report demonstrating feasibility of integration of yoga therapy in the management of urinary incontinence.

Gopal, Mondal, Gandhi, Arora, & Bhattacharjee, (2011) carried out on sixty first-year MBBS students randomly assigned to yoga group and control group (30 each). The yoga group underwent integrated yoga practices for 35 minutes daily in the presence of trained yoga teacher for 12 weeks. Control group did not undergo any kind of yoga practice or stress management. Physiological parameters like heart rate, respiratory rate, and blood pressure were measured. Global Assessment of Recent Stress Scale and Spielbergers State Anxiety score were assessed at baseline and during the examination. Serum cortisol levels, IL-4, and IFN-γ levels were determined by enzyme-linked immunosorbent assay technique. Yoga resists the autonomic changes and impairment of cellular immunity seen in examination stress

Vogler, O'Hara, Gregg, Burnell, (2011) studied with the current challenge of rapidly aging populations, practices such as yoga may help older adults stay physically active, healthy, and fulfilled. *Methods:* The impact of an 8-week Iyengar yoga program on the holistic health and well-being of physically inactive people aged 55 years and over was assessed. Thirty-eight older adults (mean age 73.21 ± 8.38 years; 19 intervention, 19 control) engaged in either twice-weekly yoga classes or continued their usual daily routines. Physical health measures were muscle strength, active range of motion, respiratory function (FEV1), resting blood pressure, and immune function (salivary IgA and lysozyme). Self-perceived general, physical, mental, spiritual, and social health and well-being were assessed with the Life's Odyssey Questionnaire and the SF12v2™ Health Survey. Participation in

Iyengar yoga programs by older people is beneficial for health and well-being, and greater availability of such programs could improve quality of life.

Shankarapillai, Nair, George, (2012) carried out in Pacific Dental College and Hospital, Udaipur, Rajasthan, India, which is a private dental school affiliated with the Rajasthan University of Health Sciences, Jaipur, India. Ethical clearance was obtained from the ethical committee and the dean of the college prior to initiating the study. Data collection took place in June 2010 in the first academic term for the year 2010-2011. The sample includes one hundred clinical undergraduate dental students (males 56%, females 44%). Given the structure of dental education at this institution, none of these students had performed a periodontal surgery procedure at the initiation of the study. One hundred clinical undergraduate dental students were invited to attend a 1-h information session about the study. All students who participated in the information session was reviewed and signed a consent form. Students then completed a baseline assessment that consisted of the demographic form (which contained the baseline VAS ratings), the STAI-trait and STAI-state. Upon completion of these baseline measures, students were randomly assigned, on an alternating basis to match the size of the groups, to Group A and Group B. Students in Group A and Group B i.e., (n=50; 28 males, 22 females; mean age 22 years) met with a researcher during a normal clinical posting separately for 60 min training. During the discussion, Group A students received a 60-min training (yoga postures *asanas*, 15 min, regulated breathing *pranayamas*, 20 min, exercises for the joints *sithilikarana vyayama*, 10 min, and guided relaxation 15 min)[24] to manage stress and anxiety while Group B received a lecture on the relation among stress, anxiety, and health. Group A received a cassette tape that contained step-by-step directions for deep breathing and was instructed to listen the tapes, practice the strategies at least once a day, and utilize the strategies as needed prior to and during their periodontal surgical procedure. Group B received cassette tapes containing ocean wave sounds, but no further instructions about how or when to use the tapes. Both groups were instructed not to tell or share information about their training with the participants in the other group. Thus, the two groups spent equivalent time with researchers in similar formats and both received audiotapes; however, Group A learned specific strategies to use to decrease anxiety and Group B did not. Most of the students stayed in single rooms and those in the shared room belonged to the same intervention group. Students of both the groups were advised to report at two recreational rooms daily at the same time to use the tape and the yoga procedure for one week. Following the 1-h training for one week, which were conducted simultaneously, varying amounts of time passed until each of the subject's first periodontal surgical procedure. The first periodontal surgical procedure was defined as the administration of local anesthetics and placement of an incision and performing a surgical procedure which need suturing for wound closure. The average span of time between the session and the procedure was 10.5 days (range=5-16 days) for Group A; likewise, this period averaged 11.5 days (range=4-15 days) for Group B. Thus, both groups averaged equally long periods of time between the initial group sessions and performing the procedure. Immediately prior to their first periodontal surgical procedure, dental student participants in both groups completed a VAS that assessed their level of anxiety and the STAI-state. A questionnaire survey was conducted among the students to assess the usefulness of the one-week session. After performing the procedure, students in both groups completed two VASs: One assessed students' level of distress and the other asked about their perception of their ability to relax. The researcher who did the statistical analysis was unaware of the grouping criteria. All the one hundred students were assessed for their general, state and expected anxiety levels using STAI-S, STAI-T and VAS. Anxiety levels were monitored at baseline, immediately prior to, and following their first periodontal surgical procedure. In this study, a significant reduction of stress was observed in Group A just prior to the performance of their first surgical procedure compared to their base line stress values. This gives them a much control over the situation and was able to relax during and after the procedure. On the other hand, Group B showed increased stress level just prior to their first surgical performance than their baseline values, which in turn affect their relaxation following the surgical procedure, i.e., they scored more on VAS and STAI-S compared to Group A. Our observations were similar to the efficacy of yogic breathing technique which was used as an anxiolytic tool in different situations.

Several studies in the medical literature showed a high incidence of stress and anxiety among medical and dental students. The institutions in the developed countries offer various counseling and stress management programs to students to cope with the situations. Among many North American medical schools, several have established policies and programs to provide treatment services and wellness programs addressing students' mental health issues. For example, following a short yoga intervention, students reported improvements in perceived stress and depressive symptoms A previous study about yogic breathing on dental students during their pediatric patient management by Piazza-Waggoner *et al.*,[14] showed no significant difference between the study and control group. He explained that during their study, a gap of 80-180 days was present between the yogic intervention and the surgical performance by students. In our study, to avoid the same error, the yogic intervention was given 5-10 days before the performance of the surgical procedure and a follow up was done during the entire clinical posting. Group A students were encouraged to do the yogic breathing immediately before the procedure. This was the main reason for the highly significant difference of anxiety levels between the groups. This study concludes that inclusion of yogic breathing in the stress reduction protocol of dental student curriculum could reduce dental students' overall anxiety, enhance their academic functioning, improve their technical performance, decrease their patients' anxiety, and ultimately benefit all aspects of their academic and professional careers. If these suggestions are implemented, the overall anxiety of dental students can be reduced, which helps them to be more successful as students, dentists and, a human being harmonious to the nature.

Cohen, Chang, Grady, & Kanaya, (2008) conducted a randomized controlled pilot trial to determine whether a restorative yoga intervention was feasible and acceptable in underactive, overweight adults with metabolic syndrome. Twenty six underactive, overweight adult men and women with metabolic syndrome were randomized to attend 15 yoga sessions of 90 minutes each over 10 weeks or to a wait-list control group. Feasibility was measured by recruitment rates, subject retention, and adherence. Acceptability was assessed by interview and questionnaires. Changes in metabolic outcomes and questionnaire measures from baseline to week 10 was calculated. Restorative yoga was a feasible and acceptable intervention in overweight adults with metabolic syndrome. The efficacy of yoga for improving metabolic parameters in this population should be explored in a larger randomized controlled trial.

Mody (2011) assessed the cardiorespiratory and metabolic responses of four rounds of Surya Namaskar, a typical amount performed by practitioners, to determine its potential as a training and weight loss tool. Six healthy Asian Indian men and women (18–22 years) who had trained in Surya Namaskar for over two years participated in the study. Testing was completed in a single session lasting about 30 min. To measure heart rate and oxygen consumption while performing the four rounds, participants were connected to a heart rate monitor and the Oxycon Mobile Metabolic System. Regular practice of Surya Namaskar may maintain or improve cardiorespiratory fitness, as well as promote weight management.

Rani, Tiwari, Singh, Agrawal, Ghildiyal, & Srivastava, (2011). To assess the impact of *Yoga Nidra* on psychological problems in patients with menstrual disorders. Patients were recruited from the Department of Obstetrics and Gynecology, C.S.M. Medical University (erstwhile KGMU), Lucknow, Uttar Pradesh, India. A total of 150 female subjects were randomly divided into two groups: 1) group of 75 subjects (with yogic intervention) and 2) a control group of 75 subjects (without yogic intervention). Assessment of psychological general wellbeing (tool) was used for all the subjects Assessment of psychological general well-being (tool) was used for all the subjects (Cases and controls). This assessment was done twice first time in the beginning (baseline) and then after six months. The current findings suggest that patients with menstrual irregularities having psychological problems improved significantly in the areas of their wellbeing, anxiety and depression by learning and applying a program based on Yogic intervention (*Yoga Nidra*).

Ankad, Herur, Patil, Shashikala, & Chinagudi, (2011) conducted to ascertain if a short-term practice of pranayama and meditation had improvements in cardiovascular functions in healthy individuals with respect to age, gender, and body mass index (BMI).This interventional study was conducted in the Department of physiology of S.N. Medical College, Bagalkot. Fifty healthy subjects (24 males and 26 females) of 20–60 years age group, fulfilling the inclusion and exclusion criteria underwent two hours daily yoga program for 15 days taught by a certified yoga teacher. Pre and post yoga cardiovascular functions were assessed by recording pulse rate, systolic blood pressure, diastolic blood pressure, and mean blood pressure.There was significant reduction in resting pulse rate, systolic blood pressure, diastolic blood pressure, and mean arterial blood pressure after practicing pranayama and meditation for 15 days. The response was similar in both the genders, both the age groups, <40 yrs and >40 yrs and both the groups with BMI, <25 kg/m^2 and >25 kg/m^2.This study showed beneficial effects of short term (15 days) regular pranayama and meditation practice on cardiovascular functions irrespective of age, gender, and BMI in normal healthy individuals.

Rao, Nagendra, Raghuram, Vinay, Chandrashekara, Gopinath, & Srinath, (2008). The aim of our study was to evaluate the effects of yoga intervention on mood states, treatment-related symptoms, quality of life and immune outcomes in breast cancer patients undergoing surgery.: Ninety-eight recently diagnosed stage II and III breast cancer patients were recruited for a randomized controlled trial comparing the effects of a yoga program with supportive therapy plus exercise rehabilitation on postoperative outcomes following surgery. Subjects were assessed prior to surgery and four weeks thereafter. Psychometric instruments were used to assess self-reported anxiety, depression, treatment-related distress and quality of life. Blood samples were collected for enumeration of T lymphocyte subsets (CD4 %, CD8 % and natural killer (NK) cell % counts) and serum immunoglobulins (IgG, IgA and IgM The results suggest possible benefits for yoga in reducing postoperative distress and preventing immune suppression following surgery

T Vadiraja, Rao, Nagarathna, Nagendra, Rekha, Vanitha, Ajaikumar, (2009) compared the effects of an integrated yoga program with brief supportive therapy in breast cancer outpatients undergoing adjuvant radiotherapy at a cancer centre. Eighty-eight stage II and III breast cancer outpatients were randomly assigned to receive yoga ($n = 44$) or brief supportive therapy ($n = 44$) prior to their radiotherapy treatment. Intervention consisted of yoga sessions lasting 60 min daily while the control group was imparted supportive therapy once in 10 days. Assessments included European Organization for Research in the Treatment of Cancer-Quality of Life (EORTCQoL C30) functional scales and Positive and Negative Affect Schedule (PANAS). Assessments were done at baseline and after 6 weeks of radiotherapy treatment. The results suggest a possible role for yoga to improve quality of life in breast cancer outpatients.

Blank, Kittel, Haberman, (2005) stated that the Iyengar system of Yoga is well suited to meet the guidelines for physical activity for breast cancer survivors. Attention to alignment and symmetry, the use of props, and careful sequencing all are improve to stamina, strength, flexibility, and confidence, while decreasing stress and side effects. Women (n = 18, ages 48 to 69 years) diagnosed with stage I–III breast cancer and receiving antiestrogen or aromatase inhibitor hormonal therapy were recruited for this study. The range of time since chemotherapy and/or radiation treatment was three months to eight years. The subjects were randomized to either a Yoga (n = 9) or wait-list control group. Beginning level Iyengar Yoga classes were conducted two times per week for eight weeks. The women were given a home instruction sheet to practice once a week at home for a total of three Yoga sessions per week. A 92.9% ± 9.8% (mean ± SD) compliance rate for weekly home practice was achieved. During the sixth week of classes, the subjects were asked to complete a 31-question self-report survey that focused on their feelings of stress, level of physical and mental effort during class sessions, and perceptions about how Yoga practice had influenced their awareness. The preliminary findings indicate that the Yoga class was well tolerated by the participants. 75% of the women reported that they would not prefer a slower paced class with less demanding poses. Yoga practice relieved the joint aches and shoulder stiffness associated with the side effects of hormonal treatment for 25% of the participants. Over 60% of the women reported improved mood and less anxiety as an outcome of the Yoga practice.

Rao, Raghuram, Nagendra, Usharani, Gopinath, Diwakar, Rao, (2015) compared the effects of yoga program with supportive therapy on self-reported symptoms of depression in breast cancer patients undergoing conventional treatment. Ninety-eight breast cancer patients with stage II and III disease from a cancer center were randomly assigned to receive yoga ($n = 45$) and supportive therapy ($n = 53$) over a 24-week period during which they underwent surgery followed by adjuvant radiotherapy (RT) or chemotherapy (CT) or both. The study stoppage criteria was progressive disease rendering the patient bedridden or any physical musculoskeletal injury resulting from intervention or less than 60% attendance to yoga intervention. Subjects underwent yoga intervention for 60 min daily with control group undergoing supportive therapy during their hospital visits. Beck's Depression Inventory (BDI) and symptom checklist were assessed at baseline, after surgery, before, during, and after RT and six cycles of CT. We used analysis of covariance (intent-to-treat) to study the effects of intervention on depression scores and Pearson correlation analyses to evaluate the bivariate relationships. The results suggest possible antidepressant effects with yoga intervention in breast cancer patients undergoing conventional treatment.

Beddoe, Lee, Weiss, Powell Kennedy, & Yang (2010) measured the effects of a mindfulness-based yoga intervention on sleep in pregnant women. Fifteen healthy, nulliparous women in their second or third trimesters with singleton pregnancies attended weekly mindfulness meditation and prenatal Hatha yoga classes in the community for 7 weeks. Sleep variables, as estimated by 72 hr of continuous wrist actigraphy and the General Sleep Disturbance Scale (GSDS), were recorded at baseline (Time 1) and postintervention (Time 2). Control data were obtained by evaluating sleep in the third-trimester group at Time 1. Due to small sample size, data were analyzed using parametric and nonparametric statistics.: Mindful yoga shows promise for women in their second trimester of pregnancy to diminish total number of awakenings at night and improve sleep efficiency and merits further exploration. Results from this pilot study provide the data to estimate sample size and design and implement powered and more controlled studies in the future.

Newham, Wittkowski, Hurley, Aplin & Westwood (2014) tested the efficacy of yoga as an intervention for reducing maternal anxiety during pregnancy.Fifty-nine primiparous, low-risk pregnant women completed questionnaires assessing state (State Trait Anxiety Inventory; STAI-State), trait (STAI-Trait), and pregnancy-specific anxiety (Wijma Delivery Expectancy Questionnaire; WDEQ) and depression (Edinburgh Postnatal Depression Scale; EPDS) before randomization (baseline) to either an 8-week course of antenatal yoga or treatment-as-usual (TAU); both groups repeated the questionnaires at follow-up. The yoga group also completed pre- and post session state anxiety and stress hormone assessments at both the first and last session of the 8-week course. Antenatal yoga seems to be useful for reducing women's anxieties toward & childbirth and preventing increases in depressive symptomatology.

Rakhshani, Nagarathna, Mhaskar, Mhaskar, Thomas & Gunasheela (2012) investigated a randomized controlled trial on the effects of yoga in prevention of pregnancy complications in high-risk pregnancies for the first time. 68 high-risk pregnant women were recruited from two maternity hospitals in Bengaluru, India and were randomized into yoga and control groups. The yoga group (n = 30) received standard care plus one-hour yoga sessions, three times a week, from the 12th to the 28th week of gestation. The control group (n = 38) received standard care plus conventional antenatal exercises (walking) during the same period. This first randomized study of yoga in high-risk pregnancy has shown that yoga can potentially be an effective therapy in reducing hypertensive related complications of pregnancy and improving fetal outcomes. Additional data is needed to confirm these results and better explain the mechanism of action of yoga in this important area.

Sun, Hung, Chang & Kuo (2010) evaluated a yoga programme provided to primigravidas in the third trimester of pregnancy with the aim of decreasing the discomforts associated with pregnancy and increasing childbirth self-efficacy. The target population was primigravidas at 26–28 weeks of gestation (no high-risk pregnancies) who had not engaged in regular exercise or yoga for at least one year. The study included 88 individuals; 43 in the control group and 45 in the experimental group who took part in the prenatal yoga programme. The duration of the prenatal yoga programme was 12–14 weeks, with at least three sessions per week. Each workout lasted for 30 minutes. The provision of booklets and videos on yoga during pregnancy may contribute to a reduction in pregnancy discomforts and improved childbirth self-efficacy.

2.3 Summary of Literature

The review of literature helped the investigator to spot out relevant topics and variables. Further, the literature helped the investigator to frame the suitable hypothesis leading to the problems. The latest literature also helped the investigator to support her findings with regard to the problem. Further the literature collected in the study will also help the research scholar understanding in the similar areas.

The reviews were presented under the study on the integrated yoga module training on physical parameter, physiological and psychological parameter with chronological order. All the research studies were presented in the section proves that there is a significant improvement on physical, physiological and psychological parameters due to integrated yoga module training.

The research studies reviewed from many journals available in the websites such as Pub Med, Science Direct Journals, ERIC websites etc., employ the physical variables such as cardio vascular endurance and muscular endurance, physiological variables such as resting pulse rate, and breath holding time and psychological variable such as stress and self-confidence.

The review of literature helped the researcher from the methodological point of view too. It was learnt that most of the research studies cited in this chapter on the integrated yoga module training would effectively improve the various physical, physiological and psychological parameter.

Chapter III

METHODOLOGY

3.1 Introduction

Research methodology involves the systematic procedure by which the researcher starts from the initial identification of the problem to its final conclusion. The role of the methodology is to carry out the research work in a scientific and valid manner.

This chapter discusses the methodology used in the selection of subjects, selection of variables, selection of tests, orientation to the subjects, competence of the tester, reliability of the instruments, reliability of the data, pilot study, training programme, collection of the data, administration of the tests, experimental design and statistical techniques were presented.

3.2 Selection of Subjects

The purpose of the study was to find out the effect of integrated yoga modules on selected physical fitness, physiological and psychological variables among Police men. To achieve the purpose of the study, thirty (N=30) Police men were selected from Tamil Nadu Special Police 9th and 12th Battalion, Manimuthar Tirunelveli District, Tamil Nadu, India. The selected subjects were randomly assigned into two groups of (n=15) each, such as experimental and control groups. Group I (n=15) underwent integrated yoga module training for a duration of 12 weeks and the number of sessions per week was confined to three alternative days, in addition to the regular training schedule

Group II (n=15) acted as control, were asked to refrain from any special training except their leisure time pursuit.

3.3 Selection of Variables

The investigator were review the available scientific literature pertaining to the study from books, journals, periodicals, magazines, research papers and available sources Manonmaniam Sundaranar University libraries and also with help of experts.

3.3.1 Dependent Variables

Physical Fitness Variables

1.   Cardio vascular endurance

2.   Muscular endurance

Physiological Variables

1.   Resting pulse rate

2.   Breath holding time

Psychological variables

1.   Stress

2.   Self Confidence

3.3.2 Independent Variables

1.   Integrated yoga modules

3.4 Selection of Tests

As per the available literature the selected variables were tested by using the following standardized tests and they were presented in Table 3.1.

Table 3.1

Selection of Tests

Sl. No	Variables	Tests / Tools	Units of Measurement
1	Cardio vascular endurance	Cooper's 12 min run and walk test	In meters
2	Muscular endurance	Sit-ups	No. of Counts per minute
3	Resting pulse Rate	Radial Pulse	Beats per minute
4	Breath holding time	Nostril clip method	In Seconds
5	Stress	Malini devi krubai 1997-Stress Inventory	In points
6	Self confidence	Rekha Agnihortry-Self Confidence inventory	In points

3.5 Orientation to the Subjects

The investigator explained the purpose of the study to the subjects and their part in the study. For the collection of the data, the investigator explained the procedure of testing on selected dependent variables and gave instructions about the procedure to be adopted by them. Four sessions were spent to familiarize the subjects with the technique involved to execute the integrated yoga modules training. It helped them to perform the given training perfectly and avoids injuries, further; the control group was specially oriented, advised and controlled to avoid the special practice of any of the specific training programme till the end of the experimental period. The participants of all the groups were sufficiently motivated to perform their maximal level during training and testing periods.

3.6 Competency of the Tester

All the measurement in this study was taken by the investigator with assistance of coach of St. John's College of Physical Education from Veeravanallur, Tirunelveli District. To ensure that the investigator and his assistance were well versed with the techniques of conducting tests, they had a number of practice sessions in the correct testing procedure. The tester's reliability was established by test and re-test method.

3.7 Reliability of the Instruments

Instruments used for this study were stop watches, sit and reach box and sphygmomanometer were availed from St. John's College of Physical Education from Veeravanallur, Tirunelveli District and purchased from reliable and standardized companies. Also, it was considered accurate enough to serve for the purpose of the study.

3.8 Reliability of the Data

Test and retest method was followed in order to establish the reliability of the data by using ten subjects at random. All the dependent variables selected in the present study were tested twice by the same personnel under similar conditions. The intra class coefficient of correlation was used to find out the reliability of the data and the results are presented in Table 3.2.

Table 3.2

Intra class co-efficient of correlation on selected variables

Sl. No	Variables	R –Value
1	Cardio vascular endurance	0.85*
2	Muscular endurance	0.85*
3	Resting pulse Rate	0.92*
4	Breath Holding Time	0.92*
5	Stress	0.88*
6	Self confidence	0.91*

*Significant at 0.01 level of confidence. (Table value required for significance at 0.01 level of confidence is 0.77)

Since the obtained 'R' values were much higher than the required value, the data were accepted as reliable in terms of instrument, tester and the subjects.

3.9 Pilot Study

Prior to the formal study sessions, a pilot study was conducted to validate research procedure and the initial capacity of the participants to design the training programme. For the purpose, 10 participants were selected at random, Group A (n=5) underwent integrated yoga modules training and group B (n=5) do not have any specific training for five sessions under the watchful eyes of the investigator. The initial loads of the participants were fixed and the training programme for group I were deigned separately based on the performance in the pilot study. While constructing the training programmes the basic principles of sports training were followed during construction of training programme, the individual differences were also considered.

3.10 Training Programme

It was a twelve week integrated yoga modules programmes for the one experimental groups at progressive intensities. Pre and post test data were collected from the experimental and control groups prior to the commencement of experiments and immediately after the training period respectively.

The duration of training session in per week three alternative days was between one hour to one and half hours approximately which included warming up and limbering down. Group II (n=15) acted as control, which did not participate in any specific training on par with experimental groups. All the subjects involved in this study were carefully monitored throughout the training programme to be away from injuries. They were questioned about their health status throughout the training programme. None of them reported with any injuries. However, muscle soreness appeared in the earlier period of the training programme and was reduced in due course.

Group I (n=15) underwent integrated yoga modules training for a duration of 12 weeks and the number of sessions per week was confined to three alternative days. The detailed training programme was presented in Appendix I, II, III.

3.11 Collection of Data

The pre and post tests data were collected on selected criterion variables prior to and immediately after the training programme among Police Men from Tamil Nadu Special Police 9th and 12th Battalion, Manimuthar, Tirunelveli District.

The tests were administered in two days in the evening sessions. The data on selected variables were tested collected by standardised test items.

3.12 Administration of Tests

3.12.1. Cardio Vascular Endurance

Purpose

The aim of this test is to measure the cardio vascular endurance (Cooper, 1968).

Equipment Required

Scorecards, electronic stopwatch, and a starting clapper.

Procedure

The subjects were positioned behind the line and upon the starting ran/ walked as many laps as possible around the track in 12 minutes. The tester and tester assistants maintained the distance covered by the subjects and when the stop signal was given by the investigator by blowing a whistle, the tester assistants ran immediately to the spot where the subject is stopped at the moment the whistle was blown. The scores were recorded in meters.

Scoring

The number of laps covered by the subject plus the number of 50 metre zone passed on the last lap within 12 minutes were measured in meters.

3.12.2. Muscular Endurance

Purpose

To measure abdominal muscular strength and endurance by performing repeated sit ups (Golding, Myers, & Sinning, 1982).

Equipment Required

Stop Watch, Whistle, Score Sheet, Paper, Pencil

Procedure

Students should lie on their backs with knees flexed, feet on floor and heels between 12 & 18 inches from the buttocks. Arms are crossed over chest with hands on opposite shoulders. Feet one held to the mat by a partner. On "Ready", "Go" the student curls to a sitting position, maintaining arm contact with chest. When elbows touch the thighs the sit-up is completed. The student then uncurls to a position where the midback contacts the mat. Students are to complete as many sit-ups in this manner as possible in one minute rest between sit-ups is allowed in either the up (or) down position.

Scoring

Only correctly performed sit-ups completed in one minute are counted.

3.12.3 Resting pulse rate

Purpose

To measure count the heart beats count of the subjects in a minutes.

Equipment

Stopwatch, stethoscope

Procedure

Resting pulse rate is calculated by the heart beat count in one minute when a player is in resting condition. The minute before taking the pulse rate the subject is asked to lie down and rest the them. The radial pulse is taken by placing three fingers on the thumb side of the wrist the pulse is counted the value in multiple by 4.

Scoring

Pulse per minute is recorded pulse rate has been recorded in beats per minutes

3.12.4. Breath Holding Time

Purpose

The purpose was to measure the ability of the subject to hold the breath for longer time.

Equipment

A stop watch with calibration of 1/10 seconds, score sheets and a pencil were used to administer this test.

Procedure

The subjects stands at ease and inhaled deeply after which he held his breath for a length of time possible to him. The index finger of the respondent served as an indicator to the Investigator to know the start and end of the recording time. The thumb and middle finger were used to hold the nose to avoid letting the air through the nostrils. The subjects were requested not to let the air out by opening the mouth while recording the breath holding time.

Scoring

The time of holding the breath till one subject let the air out was clocked by using the stop watch to the nearest one tenth of a second as breath - holding time.

3.12.5 Stress

Purpose

To assess the stress level of the subjects

Tools used

Malini devi krubai 1993 stress questionnaire was used to assess the stress

Procedure

Questionnaire describing 52 events which causes mental stress was given to the subjects and they were asked to fill yes or no along with the level of control exercised by them over event. Level of control of is assessed in three groups. Complete control, Partial control and no control.

Scoring

If the answer is Yes a score of one, two and three is assigned for complete control, partial control and no control respectively. If answer is NO then no score is assigned as the event does not bring any stress to the subject. The level is stress is arrived taking into account of the score obtained by the subject. Lower the score is considered as less stress and vice versa

Norms

Level of Stress

0 -17 Mild Stress

18 – 35 Moderate stress

36 – 52 Severe stress

Control Index

0- 51 complete control over stress

52-105 Partial control over stress

106- 156 No control over stress.

3.12.6 Self Confidence

Purpose

Agnihothri's Self-confidence Inventory (ASCI) developed by Rekha Agnihothri was used to measure self confidence.

Procedure

The ASCI questionnaire was given to all subjects. The inventory can be scored by the hand. A score of 1 ,if answered for a response indicating lack of self-confidence, that is a mark (X) to wrong response to items 2,7,23, 3 1, 40, 45, 53 and 55. On the other hand, zero score is given for responses indicated by a correct response marked (4) to the above said item.

Tools used

At the same time, for all the remaining test items above, a score of one is given for responses which are indicated by a con-ect response marked (J). On the other hand, zero is given for response indicated by a wrong response marked an (X) to all remaining items which has not been mentioned above. Lower the score the highest would be the level of self-confidence and vice versa.

3.13 Experimental Design

This study was conducted to determine possible cause and effect of integrated yoga modules on selected physical fitness, physiological and psychological variables among Police men. A pre and post test randomized control group design was employed for this investigation. This study would be consisted of two experimental group, Group-I (n=15) underwent integrated yoga modules training, and Group II (n=15) acted as control group. All the subjects were tested prior and immediately after the experimentation on selected physical fitness, physiological and psychological variables.

3.14 Statistical Technique

No attempt was made to equate the groups in any manner. Hence, to make adjustments for difference in the initial means and test the adjusted post test means for significant differences, the analysis of covariance (ANCOVA) was used **(Broota, 1989)**. All of the statistical analysis tests were computed at 0.05 level of significance (P<0.05).

3.15 Summary

Chapter 3 discussed the methods and materials used to conduct the study. The chapter began with a selection of subjects, variables and tools. The study population and sample were discussed, and the survey instrument was discussed in detail with a discussion of the rationale for choosing selected variables. Finally, data analysis, experimental design and data statistical procedures were discussed.

Chapter IV

ANALYSIS AND INTERPRETATIONS OF THE DATA

4.1 Introduction

This chapter presents the results of the study from the data analysis. The analyses were carried out through various statistical techniques such as the paired sample t-test and analysis of covariance (ANCOVA). The data were compiled and analyzed using the Statistical Package for the Social Science (SPSS) for windows computer software (Version 22).

The mode of analysis of data on the selected independent variables among the selected dependent variables has been explained in this chapter into two parts.

In part I, paired sample t-test was used to analyze the significant improvement on selected dependent variables of experimental and control group.

In part II, analysis of covariance (ANCOVA) was used to analyze the significant differences on improvement among the experimental and control groups on physical fitness, physiological and psychological variables such as cardiovascular endurance, muscular endurance, resting heart rate, breath holding time, stress and self-confidence.

Part-I

4.2 Analysis of Data for significant improvement between pre and post test of experimental and control groups on selected dependent variables

To examine if there were any statistically significant improvement of experimental and control groups on selected dependent variables.

Table 4.1 presents pre and post test means, and the results of the paired sample t-test of experimental group on selected dependent variables physical fitness, physiological and psychological variables.

Table 4.1

Paired sample 't' test of experimental group on selected dependent variables

Name of the Group	Name of the Variable	Pre Test Mean ± SD		Post Test Mean ± SD		t-test value
Experimental Group	Cardio vascular endurance	1872.33	87.91	2023.33	129.10	11.19*
	Muscular endurance	32.67	1.72	38.93	2.02	40.89*
	Resting heart rate	76.53	2.50	71.33	2.16	14.67*
	Breath holding time	38.80	1.86	47.67	2.55	23.56*
	Stress	21.33	2.02	15.47	1.77	35.51*
	Self-confidence	32.93	2.43	47.73	3.67	40.25*

*Significant of.05 level. Table value required for significant with df 14 is 2.145

The paired sample t-test was computed on selected dependent variables and the results were presented in the above Table 4.1. The 't' value for

Cardiovascular endurance is 11.19, Muscular endurance is 40.89, Resting heart rate is 14.67, Breath holding time is 23.56, Stress is 35.51 and Self-confidence is 40.25.

All the obtained 't' values are significantly higher than the required table value of 2.145 with df 14 at 0.05 level of confidence. The result of the study shows that the experimental group significantly improved the performance of all the selected dependent variables due to the 12 weeks of integrated yogic modules.

Testing of Hypothesis 1

Null hypothesis (H_0)	It was hypothesized that the experimental group would not show significant improvement on physical fitness variable as a result of the 12 week integrated yoga module.	Rejected
Researcher's hypothesis (H_1)	It was hypothesized that the experimental group would show significant improvement on physical fitness variable as a result of the 12 week integrated yoga module.	Accepted

Testing of Hypothesis 2

Null hypothesis (H_0)	It was hypothesized that the experimental group would not show significant improvement on Physiological variable as a result of the 12 week integrated yoga module.	Rejected

Researcher's hypothesis (H_1)	It was hypothesized that the experimental group would show significant improvement on physiological variable as a result of the 12 week integrated yoga module.	Accepted

Testing of Hypothesis 3

Null hypothesis (H_0)	It was hypothesized that the experimental group would not show significant improvement on psychological variable as a result of the 12 week integrated yoga module.	Rejected
Researcher's hypothesis (H_1)	It was hypothesized that the experimental group would show significant improvement on psychological variable as a result of the 12 week integrated yoga module.	Accepted

The results of the study shows that all selected physical fitness, physiological and psychological variables had significantly improved due to 12 weeks of integrated yoga module programme. Hence, the researcher's hypothesis was accepted and the null hypothesis was rejected.

Table 4.2

Paired sample 't' test of control group on selected dependent variables

Name of the Group	Name of the Variable	Pre Test Mean ± SD		Post Test Mean ± SD		t-test value
Control Group	Cardio vascular endurance	1871.25	70.98	1872.81	74.34	0.31
	Muscular endurance	32.75	1.44	33.00	2.00	1.17
	Resting heart rate	76.56	2.28	76.38	2.55	0.82
	Breath holding time	38.50	7.71	38.75	1.81	0.62
	Stress	22.06	2.21	21.94	2.35	0.62
	Self-confidence	33.50	1.75	33.63	2.09	0.49

*Significant of.05 level. Table value required for significant with df 14 is 2.145

The paired sample 't' was computed on selected dependent variables and the results were presented in the above Table 4.2. The 't' value for Cardiovascular endurance is 0.31, Muscular endurance is 1.17, Resting heart rate is 0.82, Breath holding time is 0.62, Stress is 0.62 and Self-confidence is 0.49.

All the obtained 't' test values are lesser than the required table value of 2.145 with df 14 at 0.05 level of confidence. The result of the study shows that control group had not significantly improved the selected dependent variables.

Testing of Hypothesis 4

Null hypothesis (H$_0$)	It was hypothesized that the control group would not show significant improvement between pre and post tests on physical fitness, physiological and psychological variables.	Accepted
Researcher's hypothesis (H$_1$)	It was hypothesized that the control group would show significant improvement between pre and post tests on physical fitness, physiological and psychological variables.	Rejected

The results of the study shows that all selected dependent variables such as physical fitness, physiological and psychological variables had not significantly improved. Hence, the researcher's hypothesis was rejected and the null hypothesis was accepted.

Pre-test and Post-test mean values of experimental and control groups on selected dependent variables were represented in figure 4.1 to 4.6.

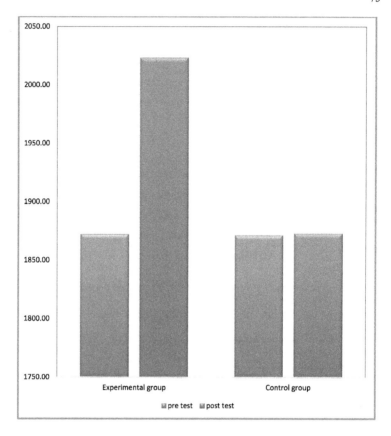

Figure 4.1

Mean values of Pre-test and post-test of cardiovascular endurance on experimental and control groups.

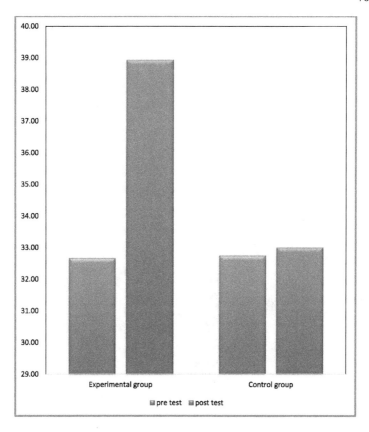

Figure 4.2

Mean values of Pre-test and post-test of Muscular endurance on experimental and control groups.

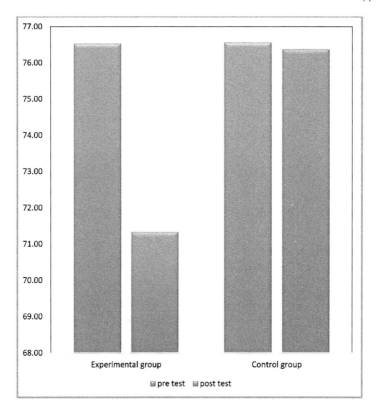

Figure 4.3

Mean values of Pre-test and post-test of resting heart rate on experimental and control groups.

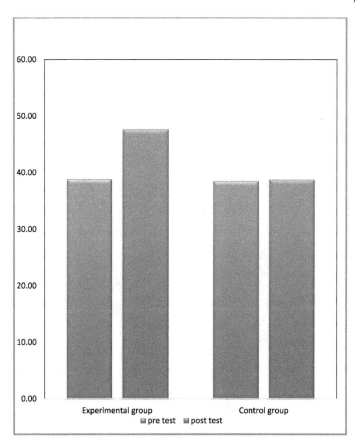

Figure 4.4

Mean values of Pre-test and post-test of breath holding time on experimental and control groups.

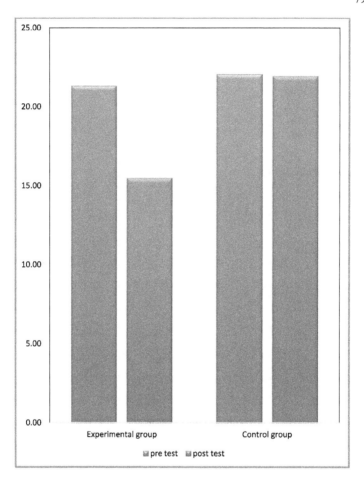

Figure 4.5

Mean values of Pre-test and post-test of Stress on experimental and control groups.

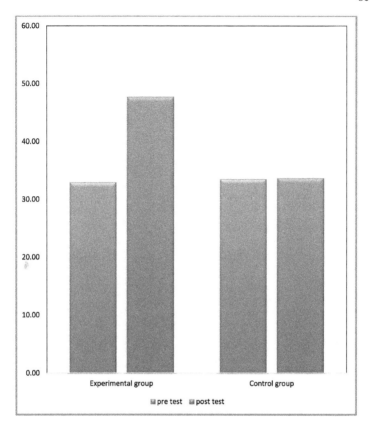

Figure 4.6

Mean values of Pre-test and post-test of Self-confidence on experimental and control groups.

Part – II

4.3 Analysis of Data for Significant Difference between experimental and control Groups on selected Dependent Variables

4.3.1 Assumptions Tests

To examine if there were any statistically significant improvement differences among the dependent variables on physical fitness, physiological and psychological variables were discussed separately.

4.3.1.1 Justifications for Using One-Way ANCOVA

One-way univariate analysis of covariance (ANCOVA) was used to determine how each dependent variable was influenced by independent variables while controlling for a covariate (pre-test) (Hari, Anderson, Tatham, and Black., 1998). Analysis of Covariance, adjusts the mean of each dependent variable to what they would be if all groups started out equally on the covariate. In this study, pretest scores of selected variables have been shown to correlate with the posttest scores, thus they were considered as appropriate covariates.

4.3.1.2 Assumptions for ANCOVA

A preliminary analysis was conducted to determine whether the prerequisite assumptions of ANCOVA were met before preceding the univariate analysis. Thus, the assumption of equality of variance (Levene's test of homogeneity), the linear regression relationship between the covariates and the dependent variables were examined.

4.3.1.3 Levene's Test

Levene's test of equality of error variances on selected variables was calculated and presented in Table 4.3.

Table 4.3

Levene's test of equality of error variances on selected dependent variables among experimental and control groups

Variables	F	df1	df2	Sig.
Cardio vascular endurance	0.06	1	29	0.81
Muscular endurance	1.06	1	29	0.31
Resting heart rate	0.06	1	29	0.81
Breath holding time	1.06	1	29	0.31
Stress	2.90	1	29	0.10
Self-confidence	0.38	1	29	0.54

(The table value required for 0.05 level of significance with df 1 & 29 is 4.18).

Homogeneity of variances is a term that is used to indicate that groups have the similar variances. Thus, in Levene's test of equality of the error variance table, the obtained F-values of the selected dependent variables were less than the confidence interval value of 0.05, which indicates that the variance of each group was not significantly different from one another. Therefore, the homogeneity of variance comparing the two groups regardless of the ability level for each of the dependent variables indicated that homogeneity of variance has been met for all the six dependent variables at significant 0.05 level of confidence. Hence, it was concluded that the assumption of homogeneity of variance has been met for computing univariate ANCOVA.

4.3.1.4 Regression of Post Test on Pre Test

The test of significance of the regression of post test (dependent variable) on pre test (covariate) were analyzed and presented in Table 4.4.

Table 4.4

Testing the significance of the regression of post test on pre test of selected dependent variables

Variables	Source of variation	Sum of Squares	df	Mean Square	F
Cardiovascular endurance	Regression	285698.42	1	285698.42	40.23*
	Residual	205938.68	29	7101.33	
Muscular endurance	Regression	94.80	1	94.80	9.33*
	Residual	294.68	29	10.16	
Resting heart rate	Regression	128.83	1	128.83	16.17*
	Residual	231.04	29	7.97	
Breath holding time	Regression	134.04	1	134.04	6.25*
	Residual	621.83	29	21.44	
Stress	Regression	184.02	1	184.02	20.00*
	Residual	266.82	29	9.20	
Self-confidence	Regression	88.49	1	88.49	4.21*
	Residual	609.26	29	21.01	

* Significant at 0.05 level of confidence (The table value required for 0.05 level of significance with df 1and 29 is 4.18).

From the Table 4.4 it was observed that regression based method (ANCOVA) predicts the post test scores significantly well from the pre test scores on all the dependent variables at significant 0.05 level of confidence. Hence, it was concluded that the linear regression relationship between the covariates has been met for computing univariate ANCOVA. It shows that the pre and post test scores of selected dependent variables were significantly associated. As in regression, it is important that the association between the outcome and the covariate is linear.

4.3.2 Results of Analysis of Covariance (ANCOVA)

4.3.2.1 Cardio vascular Endurance

The results of the univariate ANCOVA for experimental and control group on cardio vascular endurance was presented in table 4.5.

Table 4.5

Analysis of covariance computed for experimental and control group for cardio vascular endurance

Variable	Adjusted post mean		Sum of Squares	df	Mean Square	F
	Experimental group	Control group				
Cardiovascular endurance	2022.64	1873.46	172279.89	1	172279.89	143.32*
			33658.79	28	1202.10	

*Significant at .05 level. Table value required for significance at 0.05 level with df 1 and 28 was 4.20.

Analysis of covariance (ANCOVA) was computed for cardiovascular endurance. The independent variables included one training groups, namely experimental group. The dependent variable was cardiovascular endurance and the covariate was an initial performance of the cardiovascular endurance. The 'F' ratio was significant for df $(1, 28) = 143.32$, p <0.05 (See Table 4.5). It shows that the experimental group had significant difference on cardiovascular endurance when compared to control group.

Testing of Hypothesis 5 on Cardiovascular Endurance

Researcher's hypothesis (H_1)	It was also hypothesized that the experimental group had significant difference when compare to control group in cardiovascular endurance than a control group.	Accepted
Null hypothesis (H_0)	It was also hypothesized that the experimental group had significant difference when compare to control group in cardiovascular endurance than a control group.	Rejected

Figure 4.7 illustrates the adjusted post test means of experimental and control groups on Cardio respiratory endurance.

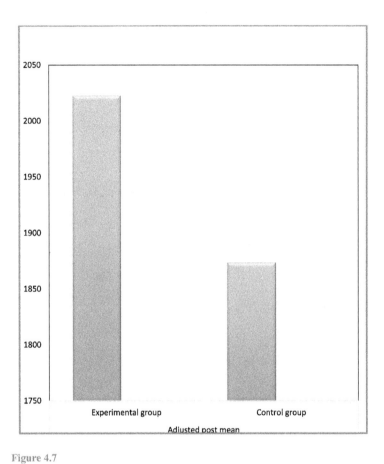

Figure 4.7

Adjusted post test mean values of Experimental group and control group on cardio vascular endurance.

4.3.2.2 Muscular Endurance

The results of the univariate ANCOVA for experimental and control group on muscular endurance was presented in table 4.6.

Table 4.6

Analysis of covariance computed for experimental and control group for muscular endurance

Variable	Adjusted post mean		Sum of Squares	df	Mean Square	F
	Experimental group	Control group				
Muscular endurance	38.99	32.95	281.59	1	281.59	602.193*
			13.09	28	0.47	

*Significant at .05 level. Table value required for significance at 0.05 level with df 1 and 28 was 4.20.

One way analysis of covariance (ANCOVA) was computed for muscular endurance. The independent variables included one training groups, namely experimental group. The dependent variable was muscular endurance and the covariate was an initial performance of the muscular endurance. The ANCOVA 'F' ratio was significant for df $(1, 28) = 602.193$, $p < 0.05$ (See Table 4.6). It shows that the experimental group had significant improvement difference on muscular endurance when compared to control group

Figure 4.8 illustrates the adjusted post test means of experimental and control groups on Muscular endurance.

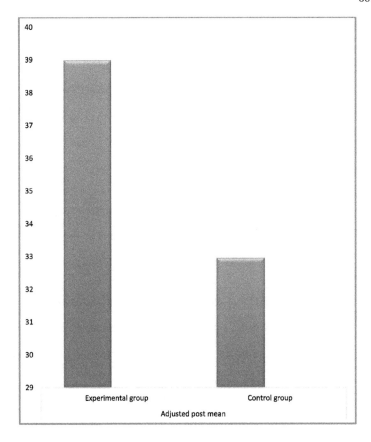

Figure 4.8

Adjusted post test mean values of Experimental group and control group on muscular endurance.

Testing of Hypothesis 3 on muscular endurance

Researcher's hypothesis (H_1)	It was also hypothesized that the experimental group had significant difference when compare to control group in muscular endurance than a control group.	Accepted
Null hypothesis (H_0)	It was also hypothesized that the experimental group had significant difference when compare to control group in muscular endurance than a control group.	Rejected

The results of the study shows that selected dependent variable muscular endurance has shows that significant difference between the experimental and control group due to the 12 week integrated yoga module training programs. Hence, the researcher's hypothesis were accepted and the null hypothesis was rejected.

4.3.2.3 Resting Pulse Rate

The results of the univariate ANCOVA for experimental and control group on resting pulse rate was presented in table 4.7.

Table 4.7

Analysis of covariance computed for experimental and control group for resting pulse rate

Variable	Adjusted post mean		Sum of Squares	df	Mean Square	F
	Experimental group	Control group				
Resting pulse rate	71.35	76.36	194.79	1	194.79	150.47*
			36.25	28	1.30	

*Significant at .05 level. Table value required for significance at 0.05 level with df 1 and 28 was 4.20.

One way analysis of covariance (ANCOVA) was computed for resting pulse rate. The independent variables included one training groups, namely experimental group. The dependent variable was muscular endurance and the covariate was an initial performance of the resting pulse rate. The ANCOVA 'F' ratio was significant for df $(1, 28) = 150.47$, p <0.05 (See Table 4.6). It shows that the experimental group had significant improvement difference on resting pulse rate when compared to control group.

Figure 4.9 illustrates the adjusted post test means of experimental and control groups on resting pulse rate.

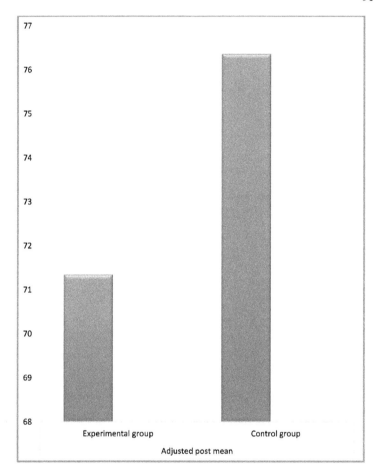

Figure 4.9

Adjusted post test mean values of Experimental group and control group on resting pulse rate.

Testing of Hypothesis 5 on resting pulse rate

Researcher's hypothesis (H_1)	It was also hypothesized that the experimental group had significant difference when compare to control group in resting pulse rate than a control group.	Accepted
Null hypothesis (H_0)	It was also hypothesized that the experimental group had significant difference when compare to control group in resting pulse rate than a control group.	Rejected

The results of the study shows that selected dependent variable resting pulse rate has shows that significant difference between the experimental and control group due to the 12 week integrated yoga module training programs. Hence, the researcher's hypothesis was accepted and the null hypothesis was rejected.

4.3.2.4 Breath Holding Time

The results of the univariate ANCOVA for experimental and control group on breath holding time was presented in table 4.8.

Table 4.8

Analysis of covariance computed for experimental and control group for Breath Holding Time

Variable	Adjusted post mean		Sum of Squares	df	Mean Square	F
	Experimental group	Control group				
Breath holding time	47.51	38.89	571.115	1	571.115	315.33*
			50.71	28	1.81	

*Significant at .05 level. Table value required for significance at 0.05 level with df 1 and 47 was 4.20.

One way analysis of covariance (ANCOVA) was computed for throwing ability. The independent variables included one training groups, namely experimental group. The dependent variable was throwing and the covariate was an initial performance of the throwing ability. The ANCOVA 'F' ratio was significant for df $(1, 28) = 315.33$, p <0.05 (See Table 4.8). It shows that the experimental group had significant improvement difference on Breath Holding Time when compared to control group.

Figure 4.10 illustrates the adjusted post test means of experimental and control groups on Breath holding time.

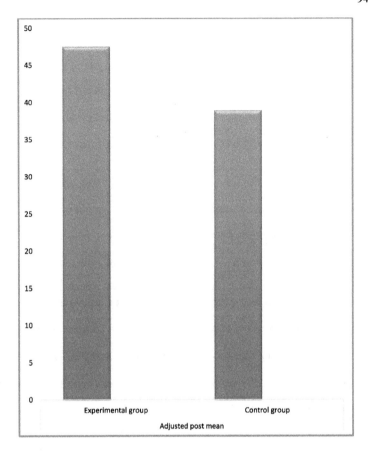

Figure 4.10

Adjusted post test mean values of Experimental group and control group on breath holding time.

Testing of Hypothesis 5 on breath holding time

Researcher's hypothesis (H_1)	It was also hypothesized that the experimental group had significant difference when compare to control group in breath holding time than a control group.	Accepted
Null hypothesis (H_0)	It was also hypothesized that the experimental group had significant difference when compare to control group in breath holding time than a control group.	Rejected

The results of the study shows that selected dependent variable breath holding time has shows that significant difference between the experimental and control group due to the 12 week integrated yoga module training programs. Hence, the researcher's hypothesis was accepted and the null hypothesis was rejected.

4.3.2.5 Stress

The results of the univariate ANCOVA for experimental and control group on stress was presented in table 4.9.

Table 4.9

Analysis of covariance computed for experimental and control group for Stress

Variable	Adjusted post mean		Sum of Squares	df	Mean Square	F
	Experimental group	Control group				
Stress	15.82	21.61	252.03	1	252.03	477.32*
			14.78	28	0.53	

*Significant at .05 level. Table value required for significance at 0.05 level with df 1 and 28 was 4.20

One way analysis of covariance (ANCOVA) was computed for stress. The independent variables included one training groups, namely experimental group. The dependent variable was stress and the covariate was an initial performance of the stress. The ANCOVA 'F' ratio was significant for df (1, 28) = 477.32, p <0.05 (See Table 4.9). It shows that the experimental group had significant improvement difference on stress when compared to control group.

Figure 4.11 illustrates the adjusted post test means of experimental and control groups on Stress.

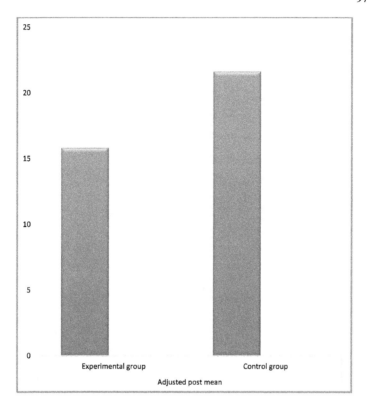

Figure 4.11

Adjusted post test mean values of Experimental group and control group on Stress.

Testing of Hypothesis 5 on stress

Researcher's hypothesis (H_1)	It was also hypothesized that the experimental group had significant difference when compare to control group in stress than a control group.	Accepted
Null hypothesis (H_0)	It was also hypothesized that the experimental group had significant difference when compare to control group in stress than a control group.	Rejected

The results of the study shows that selected dependent variable stress has shows that significant difference between the experimental and control group due to the 12 week specific motor skill training programs. Hence, the researcher's hypothesis was accepted and the null hypothesis was rejected.

4.3.2.6 Self-Confidence

The results of the univariate ANCOVA for experimental and control group on self confidence was presented in table 4.10.

Table 4.10

Analysis of covariance computed for experimental and control group for Self Confidence

Variable	Adjusted post mean		Sum of Squares	df	Mean Square	F
	Experimental group	Control group				
Self confidence	48.12	33.26	89.84	1	1675.95	1502.17*
			23.28	28	1.116	

*Significant at .05 level. Table value required for significance at 0.05 level with df 1 and 28 was 4.20.

One way analysis of covariance (ANCOVA) was computed for self-confidence. The independent variables included one training groups, namely experimental group. The dependent variable was self-confidence and the covariate was an initial performance of the self-confidence. The ANCOVA 'F' ratio was significant for df (1, 28) = 1502.17, p <0.05 (See Table 4.10). It shows that the experimental group had significant improvement difference on self-confidence when compared to control group.

Figure 4.12 illustrates the adjusted post test means of experimental and control groups on Self-Confidence.

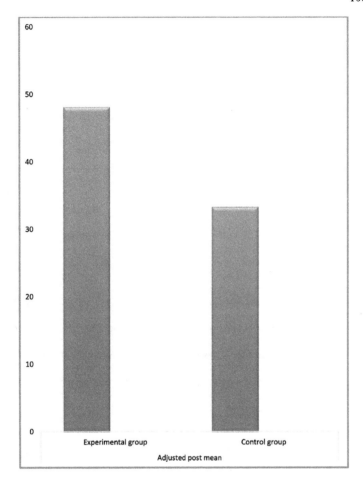

Figure 4.12

Adjusted post test mean values of Experimental group and control group on Self-confidence.

Testing of Hypothesis 3 on self confidence

Researcher's hypothesis (H_1)	It was also hypothesized that the experimental group had significant difference when compare to control group in self confidence than a control group.	Accepted
Null hypothesis (H_0)	It was also hypothesized that the experimental group had significant difference when compare to control group in self confidence than a control group.	Rejected

The results of the study shows that selected dependent variable self confidence has shows that significant difference between the experimental and control group due to the 12 week integrated yoga module training programs. Hence, the researcher's hypothesis was accepted and the null hypothesis was rejected.

4.4 Discussion on Findings

The result of the study indicated that,

4.4.1 Physical fitness

The experimental group had achieved significant improvement on physical fitness variables such as cardiovascular endurance and muscular endurance due to the effect of integrated yoga module training.

Also there is a significance improvement difference between experimental and control group on physical fitness variables such as cardiovascular endurance and muscular endurance.

4.4.2 Physiological

The experimental group had achieved significant improvement on physiological variables such as resting heart rate and breath holding timedue to the effect of integrated yoga module training.

Also there is a significance improvement difference between experimental and control group on physiological variables such as resting heart rate and breath holding time.

4.4.3 Psychological

The experimental group had achieved significant improvement on Psychological variables such as stress and self-confidencedue to the effect of integrated yoga module training.

Also there is a significance improvement difference between experimental and control group on Psychological variables such as stress and self-confidence.

4.4.4 Supported studies

The findings of the present study were supported by the limited literature suggesting that physical fitness, physiological and psychological can have positive impact on integrated yoga module Amaranath, Nagendra, & Deshpande, (2016) study the efficacy of integrated *Yoga* module on emotions (positive and negative affect) of Home guards. The results suggested that IYM can be useful for HGs to improve the Positive affect and to decrease negative affect score. Moreover, integrated *Yoga* module is cost-effective and helps HGs for coping up with emotions in stressful situations.

Patil, Mullur, Khodnapur, Dhanakshirur, & Aithala, (2013) aimed to evaluate the effect of integrated yoga module on heart rate variability (HRV) measure as a stress index in sub junior cyclists.In conclusion, yoga practice helps to reduce stress byoptimizing the autonomic functions. So, it is suggested to incorporateyoga module as a regular feature to keep subjunior athletes both mentallyand physically fit.

Choukse, Ram, & Nagendra, (2018) conducted the effect of residential integrated yoga on physical fitness of adolescents using eurofit battery.

Sethi, Nagendra, & Ganpat, (2013) assessed attention and SE in girls undergoing Integrated Yoga Module. The present study suggests that of IYM can result in improvement of attention and SE among students.

Chapter V

SUMMARY, CONCLUSIONS AND RECOMMENDATIONS

5.1 Summary

This chapter discussed about the obtained results from the chapter IV and frame the conclusion and recommendation.

The purpose of the study was to find out the effect of integrated yoga modules on selected physical fitness, physiological and psychological variables among Police men. To achieve the purpose of the study, thirty (N=30) Police men were selected from Tamil Nadu Special Police 9th and 12th Battalion, Manimuthar Tirunelveli District, Tamil Nadu, India. The selected subjects were randomly assigned into two groups of (n=15) each, such as experimental and control groups. Group I (n=15) underwent integrated yoga modules training for a duration of 12 weeks and the number of sessions per week was confined to three alternative days, in addition to the regular schedule of the curriculum. Group II (n=15) acted as control, were asked to refrain from any special training except their leisure time pursuit as college students.

The following dependent variables were selected for this study such as Physical fitness (cardiovascular endurance and muscular endurance), Physiological variable (resting heart rate and breath holding time) and Psychological variable (stress and self-confidence).

The pre test and post-test randomized control group design was employed for this investigation. The thirty participants are divided into two groups, Group I (n=15) underwent integrated yoga module, and Group II (n=15) acted as control group. The collected data from the two groups prior to and immediately after the training programme on selected criterion variables were statistically analyzed with paired sample 't' test to find out the significant improvement between pre and post-test means and analysis of covariance (ANCOVA) was used to find out the significance difference between experimental and control groups. In all the cases 0.05 level of significant was fixed to test the hypothesis.

5.2 Conclusions

1. There was a significant improvement among experimental group on cardiovascular endurance due to the effect of 12 week of integrated yoga module.

2. There was a significant improvement among experimental group on muscular endurance due to the effect of 12 week of integrated yoga module.

3. There was a significant improvement among experimental group on resting pulse rate due to the effect of 12 week of integrated yoga module.

4. There was a significant improvement among experimental group on breath holding time due to the effect of 12 week of integrated yoga module.

5. There was a significant improvement among experimental group on stress due to the effect of 12 week of integrated yoga module.

6. There was a significant improvement on among experimental group Self-confidence due to the effect of 12 week of integrated yoga module.

7. There was no significant improvement among control group on cardiovascular endurance due to the effect of 12 week of integrated yoga module.

8. There was no significant improvement among control group on muscular endurance due to the effect of 12 week of integrated yoga module.

9. There was no significant improvement among control group on resting pulse rate due to the effect of 12 week of integrated yoga module.

10. There was no significant improvement among control group on breath holding time due to the effect of 12 week of integrated yoga module.

11. There was no significant improvement among control group on stress due to the effect of 12 week of integrated yoga module.

12. There was no significant improvement among control group Self-confidence due to the effect of 12 week of integrated yoga module.

13. There was a significant difference between the experimental and control groups in improving the physical fitness variables such as cardio vascular endurance and muscular endurance.

14. There was a significant difference between the experimental and control groups in improving the physiological variables such as resting heart rate and breath holding time.

15. There was a significant difference between the experimental and control groups in improving the psychological variables such as stress and self-confidence.

5.3 Recommendations for Future Researchers

1. A limitation of this study was the lack of follow-up procedures. It still remains to be determined if the fitness status improvements gained from instruction were maintained over time. Future research should attempt to longitudinally to study the policeman receiving such instruction.

2. Future research is needed to evaluate the body compositions completely with long-term follow-up.

3. Future research is needed to evaluate the bio motor variables completely with long-term follow-up.

4. Future research is needed to evaluate the bio chemical components completely with long-term follow-up.

5. The similar study may be conducted by selecting larger sample with over a period of time among Tamil Nadu police people.

6. The comparison of gender and age group may be studied along with physical and mental aspects intervention programme.

References

Amaranath B1, Nagendra HR1, Deshpande S1.Department of Yoga and Life Science, S-VYASA Yoga University, Bengaluru, Karnataka, India. Int J Yoga. 2016 Jan-Jun; 9(1):35-43. doi: 10.4103/0973-6131.171719.

Amaranath B1, Nagendra HR2, Deshpande S2.Yoga & Life Science, S-VYASA Yoga University, Bengaluru, Karnataka, India. Electronic address: b_amaranath@yahoo.co.in.Yoga & Life Science, S-VYASA Yoga University, Bengaluru, Karnataka, India. J Ayurveda Integr Med. 2016 Mar;7(1):44-7. doi: 10.1016/j.jaim.2015.11.002. Epub 2016 May 24.

Amaranath, B. (2015). Effect Of Integrated Yoga Module On Emotions Personality Stress Verbal Aggression And Satisfaction With Life Of Home Guards In Bangalore.

Amaranath, B., Nagendra, H. R., & Deshpande, S. (2016). Effect of integrated Yoga module on positive and negative emotions in Home Guards in Bengaluru: A wait list randomized control trial. International journal of yoga, 9(1), 35.

Amaranath, B., Nagendra, H. R., & Deshpande, S. (2016). Effect of integrated Yoga module on positive and negative emotions in Home Guards in Bengaluru: A wait list randomized control trial. International journal of yoga, 9(1), 35.

Amaranath, B., Nagendra, H. R., & Deshpande, S. (2016). Effect of integrated yoga module on personality of home guards in Bengaluru: A randomized control trial. Journal of Ayurveda and integrative medicine, 7(1), 44-47.

Balakrishnan, R., Nanjundaiah, R. M., Nirwan, M., Sharma, M. K., Ganju, L., Saha, M., ... & Ramarao, N. H. (2019). Design and validation of Integrated Yoga Therapy module for Antarctic expeditioners. Journal of Ayurveda and integrative medicine.

Baumgartner, T. A., & Jackson, A. S. (1991). Measurement for evaluation in physical education and exercise science. Dubuque: Wm. C. C. Publishers.

Bhavanani, A. B. (2011). Understanding the science of yoga. Int. Yoga Scientif. J. SENSE, 1, 334-344.

Bhavanani, A. B., Udupa, K., & Madanmohan, P. N. (2011). A comparative study of slow and fast suryanamaskar on physiological function. International journal of yoga, 4(2), 71.

Bhutkar, P. M., Bhutkar, M. V., Taware, G. B., Doijad, V., & Doddamani, B. R. (2008). Effect of suryanamaskar practice on cardio-respiratory fitness parameters: A pilot study. Al Ameen J Med Sci, 1(2), 126-129.

Bjlani RL.(2004). Understanding medical physiology; 3rd ed. New Delhi: Jaypee Brothers; pp. 871–910

Chen, K. M., & Tseng, W. S. (2008). Pilot-testing the effects of a newly-developed silver yoga exercise program for female seniors. Journal of Nursing Research, 16(1), 37-46.

Chobe S, Bhargav H, Raghuram N, Garner C. J Complement Integr Med (2016) Sep 1;13(3):301-309. doi: 10.1515/jcim-2015-0105.

Choudhary, R., & Stec, K. (2010). The effect of dynamic Suryanamaskar on flexibility of university students. JAD Research, 1(1), 45-48.

Choukse, A., Ram, A., & Nagendra, H. R. (2018). Effect of residential integrated yoga on physical fitness of adolescents using eurofit battery

Cooper, K. H. (1968). A means of assessing maximal oxygen intake: correlation between field and treadmill testing. Jama, 203(3), 201-204.

Datey, K. K., & Gharote, M. S. (1985) Yoga for your heart: Jaico Publishing house. Mumbai, pg, 11-15.

Ebnezar, J., Nagarathna, R., Yogitha, B., & Nagendra, H. R. (2012). Effect of integrated yoga therapy on pain, morning stiffness and anxiety in osteoarthritis of the knee joint: A randomized control study. International Journal of Yoga, 5(1), 28.

Ebnezar, J., Nagarathna, R., Yogitha, B., & Nagendra, H. R. (2012). Effects of an integrated approach of hatha yoga therapy on functional disability, pain, and flexibility in osteoarthritis of the knee joint: a randomized controlled study. The Journal of Alternative and Complementary Medicine, 18(5), 463-472.

Feuerstein, G. (1998). The yoga tradition: It's history, literature, philosophy, and practice. Prescott, AZ: Hohm Press.

Ganpat TS1, Nagendra HR.Department of Yoga and Management, Swami Vivekananda Yoga Anusandhana Samsthana University, Prashanti Kutiram, Bangalore, Karnataka, India. Ind Psychiatry J. 2011 Jan;20(1):45-8. doi: 10.4103/0972-6748.98415.

Gnanabakthan, J. (2011). Effects of different packages of yogic practices on selected health fitness components physiological and psychological variables among police men in Chennai.

Golding, L. A., Myers, C. R., & Sinning, W. E. (Eds.). (1982). Y's way to physical fitness. YMCA of the USA.

Kakde, N., Metri, K. G., Varambally, S., Nagaratna, R., & Nagendra, H. R. (2017). Development and validation of a yoga module for Parkinson disease. Journal of Complementary and Integrative Medicine, 14(3).

Karvonen, M. J. (1957). The effects of training on heart rate: a longitudinal study. Ann Med Exp Biol Fenn, 35, 307-315.

Lokeswarananda, S., & Taittiriya, U. (1996) Calcutta: Ramakrishna Mission Institute of Culture; The Ramakrishna Mission Institute of Culture, 136-80.

MacMahon, S. W., Blacket, R. B., Macdonald, G. J., & Hall, W. (1984). Obesity, alcohol consumption and blood pressure in Australian men and women. The National Heart Foundation of Australia Risk Factor Prevalence Study. Journal of hypertension, 2(1), 85-91.

Maharana, S., Nagarathna, R., Padmalatha, V., Nagendra, H. R., & Hankey, A. (2013). The effect of integrated yoga on labor outcome: A randomized controlled study. International Journal of Childbirth, 3(3), 165-177.

Mahatma Gandhi Medical College and Research Institute, Puducherry, 607402 West Indian Med J. 2014 Jan; 63(1): 78–80.Published online 2014 Nov 25. doi: 10.7727/wimj.2012.054

Mandlik, V. (2001). Yog Shikshan Mala, Yog Parichay.

Malini devi kirubai, family structure in relation to stress coping of general heath of women, inpublished M. phil Dissertation, university of madras, 1993.

Mealey, M. (1979). New fitness for police and fire fighters. The Physician and sportsmedicine, 7(7), 96-100.

Moghe, G. L. (2015). A Study Of Effect Of Selected Yogic Practices And The Problems During Menopausal Period Of Women Between 35 To 60 Age Group.

Morehouse, L. E., & Miller, A. T. (1967). Physiology ofexercise. St Louis: Mosby.

Nagarathna, R., & Nagendra, H. R. (2003). Integrated approach of yoga therapy for positive health. Swami Vivekananda Yoga Prakashana. Bangalore, India, 20011.

Nagendra, H. R. (2015). Effect of Integrated Yoga Module on Perceived Stress, Verbal Aggression and Satisfaction with Life in Home Guards in Bangalore–A Wait List Randomized Control Trial. Journal of Ayurveda and Holistic Medicine (JAHM), 3(5), 21-38.

Nambinarayanan, T., Thakur, S., Krishnamurthy, N., & Chandrabose, A. (1992). Effect of yoga training on reaction time, respiratory endurance and muscle strength. Indian J Physiol Pharmacol, 36(4), 229-233.

Naoroibam, R., Metri, K. G., Bhargav, H., Nagaratna, R., & Nagendra, H. R. (2016). Effect of Integrated Yoga (IY) on psychological states and CD4 counts of HIV-1 infected Patients: A Randomized controlled pilot study. International journal of yoga, 9(1), 57.

Naranjo, C., & Ornstein, R. E. (1971). On the psychology of meditation. Viking Adult.

Narasimhan L, Nagarathna R, Nagendra H. (2011) Division of Life Sciences and Yoga, Swami Vivekananda Yoga Aunsandhana Samsthana (SVYASA), Jigani, Bangalore, Karnataka, India. Int J Yoga. Jan;4(1):13-9. doi: 10.4103/0973-6131.78174

Narasimhan, L., Nagarathna, R., & Nagendra, H. R. (2011). Effect of integrated yogic practices on positive and negative emotions in healthy adults. International journal of yoga, 4(1), 13.

Naveen GH1, Rao MG, Vishal V, Thirthalli J, Varambally S, Gangadhar BN.Department of Psychiatry, National Institute of Mental Health and Neuro Sciences, Bangalore, Karnataka, India2013 Jul;55(Suppl 3):S350-6. doi: 10.4103/0019-5545.116305..

Parthasarathy, S., & Jaiganesh, K. (2014). Effect of integrated yoga module on selected psychological variables among women with anxiety problem. West Indian Medical Journal, 63(1), 78-80.

Patil NJ, Nagarathna R, Tekur P, Patil DN, Nagendra HR, Subramanya P, .Department of Integrative Medicine, Sri Devaraj Urs University, Tamka, Kolar, Karnataka, India.Division of Yoga and Life Sciences, S-VYASA Yoga University, Bengaluru, Karnataka, India2015 Jul-Dec;8(2):103-8.

Patil, N. J., Nagarathna, R., Tekur, P., Patil, D. N., Nagendra, H. R., & Subramanya, P. (2015). Designing, validation, and feasibility of integrated yoga therapy module for chronic low back pain. International journal of yoga, 8(2), 103.

Patil, S. S. (2014). Efficacy Of Integrated Yoga Module On Prakrti Of The Children.

Pise V1, Pradhan B1, Gharote MM2.Swami Vinvekanada Yoga Anusandhan Samsthan University (SVYASA), Eknath Bhavan, Bengaluru, Karnataka, India.Lonavla Yoga Institute, Pune, Maharashtra, India. 2017 Jul-Dec;26 (2):151-154.

Pise, V., Pradhan, B., & Gharote, M. M. (2017). Validation of yoga module for children with intellectual disabilities. Industrial psychiatry journal, 26(2), 151.

Rakhshani, A., Maharana, S., Raghuram, N., Nagendra, H. R., & Venkatram, P. (2010). Effects of integrated yoga on quality of life and interpersonal relationship of pregnant women. Quality of Life Research, 19(10), 1447-1455.

Ram A, Raghuram N, Rao RM, Bhargav H, Koka PS, Tripathi S, Nelamangala RV, Kodaganur GS, Ramarao NH. J Stem Cells. 2012;7(4):269-82. doi: jsc.2013.7.4.269.

Rao, K. R. (1989). Meditation: Secular and sacred: A review and assessment of some recent research. Journal of the Indian Academy of Applied Psychology.

Rathi, S. S., Raghuaram, N., Tekur, P., Joshi, R. R., & Ramarao, N. H. (2018). Development and validation of integrated yoga module for obesity in adolescents. International journal of yoga, 11(3), 231.

Rekha agnithory. " Manual for agnithotri self confidence inventory (ASCI) " (psychological corporation),agra,1987.p.2-3

Rshikesan PB1, Subramanya P2.Research Scholar, Division of Yoga and Life Sciences, Swami Vivekananda Yoga Anusandhana Samsthana , Bengaluru, Karnataka, India .Associate Professor, Division of Yoga and Life Sciences, 19 S- VYASA Yoga University , Gavipuram Circle, K.G. Nagar, Bengaluru, Karnataka, India . J Clin Diagn Res. 2016 Oct;10(10):KC01-KC06. Epub 2016 Oct 1.

Rshikesan, P. B., & Subramanya, P. (2016). Effect of Integrated Approach of Yoga Therapy on Male Obesity and Psychological Parameters-A Randomised Controlled Trial. Journal of clinical and diagnostic research: JCDR, 10(10), KC01.

S Parthasarathy,1 K Jaiganesh,1 and Duraisamy2 Effect of Integrated Yoga Module on Selected Psychological Variables among Women with Anxiety Problem

Saraswati, S. S. (1996). Surya namaskara: a technique of solar vitalization. Bihar School of Yoga.

Satyapriya, M., Nagarathna, R., Padmalatha, V., & Nagendra, H. R. (2013). Effect of integrated yoga on anxiety, depression & well being in normal pregnancy. Complementary therapies in clinical practice, 19(4), 230-236.

Satyapriya, M., Nagarathna, R., Padmalatha, V., & Nagendra, H. R. (2013). Effect of integrated yoga on anxiety, depression & well being in normal pregnancy. Complementary therapies in clinical practice, 19(4), 230-236.

Satyapriya, M., Nagendra, H. R., Nagarathna, R., & Padmalatha, V. (2009). Effect of integrated yoga on stress and heart rate variability in pregnant women. International Journal of Gynecology & Obstetrics, 104(3), 218-222.

Sethi, J. K., Nagendra, H. R., & Ganpat, T. S. (2013). Yoga improves attention and self-esteem in underprivileged girl student. Journal of education and health promotion, 2.

Sinha, B., Ray, U. S., Pathak, A., & Selvamurthy, W. (2004). Energy cost and cardiorespiratory changes during the practice of Surya Namaskar. Indian journal of physiology and pharmacology, 48(2), 184-190.

Sjoman, N. E. (1999). The yoga tradition of the Mysore Palace. Abhinav publications.

Smolander, J., Louhevaaral, V., & Oja, P. (1984). Policemen's physical fitness in relation to the frequency of leisure-time physical excercise. International archives of occupational and environmental health, 54(4), 295-302.

Snyder, C. R., & Lopez, S. J. (Eds.). (2009). Oxford handbook of positive psychology. Oxford library of psychology.

Solberg, E. E., Halvorsen, R., Sundgot-Borgen, J., Ingjer, F., & Holen, A. (1995). Meditation: a modulator of the immune response to physical stress? A brief report. British Journal of Sports Medicine, 29(4), 255-257.

Swami Shri Shiwanand Saraswati, 'Pranayam: A Science' 8th Ed, (Ahmedabad: Shivanand Science Nidhi Divya Jivan Sangh

Swaminathan, S., Venkatesan, P., & Mukunthan, R. (1993). Peack expiratory flow rate in South Indian Children. Indian pediatrics, 30(2), 207-211.

Tamil Nadu Police Archives October 24, 2007, at the Wayback Machine

Telles, S., Hanumanthaiah, B., Nagarathna, R., & Nagendra, H. R. (1993). Improvement in static motor performance following yogic training of school children. Perceptual and Motor Skills, 76(3_suppl), 1264-1266.

US RAY, S. M., Purkayastha, S., ASNANI, V., Tomer, O., PRASHAD, R., THAKUR, L., & Selvamurthy, W. (2001). Effect of yogic exercises on physical and mental health of young fellowship course trainees. Indian J Physiol Pharmacol, 45(1), 37-53.

Verma, Bhargav, Varambally, Raghuram, & Gangadhar, (2018). Effect of integrated yoga on anti-psychotic induced side effects and cognitive functions in patients suffering from schizophrenia. Journal of Complementary and Integrative Medicine, 16 (1).

Walter, C. (1932). The wisdom of the body.

Wells, K. F., & Dillon, E. K. (1952). The sit and reach—a test of back and leg flexibility. Research Quarterly. American Association for Health, Physical Education and Recreation, 23(1), 115-118.

West, J., Otte, C., Geher, K., Johnson, J., & Mohr, D. C. (2004). Effects of Hatha yoga and African dance on perceived stress, affect, and salivary cortisol. Annals of Behavioral Medicine, 28(2), 114-118.

White, David Gordon (2014), The "Yoga Sutra of Patanjali": A Biography, Princeton University Press.

CPSIA information can be obtained
at www.ICGtesting.com
Printed in the USA
BVHW051803231222
654915BV00010B/1115